My Connections Magazine

Table of Content:

I0419198

ON THE COVER

TIME IS MONEY

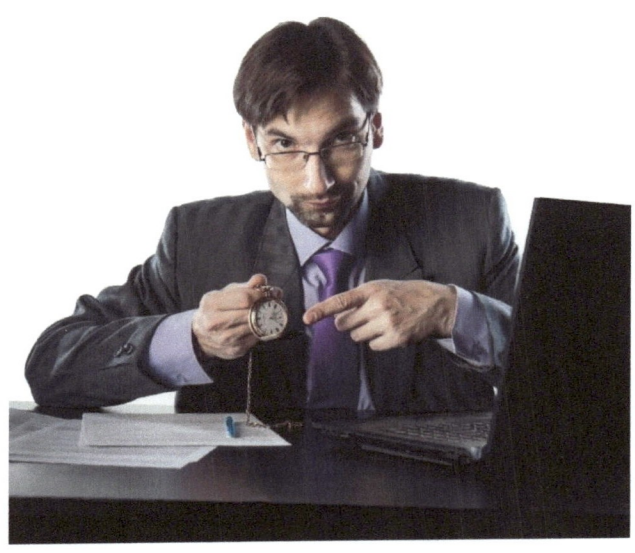

How can you tell that time is money? Try to get a job, hire a cab, ask what does it cost of anything you purchase, and immediately you hear labor added to the French fries you just eat, and why you have to pay more this time for your short Taxi trip to your doctor. Increase in wages mean it is going to cost you. Wages are disbursed per hour in most jobs, others are called salaries and are paid per month although the overall wages are calculated in total hours must be worked during the month.

In long term time is money can be related to college graduation and a degree completion on time, otherwise one can be losing on both side of the college wall. Time is money in overtime, deadline, and many other projects that are paid by using time frame.

But the term 'time is money" used alone to refer to the loss of money by wasting time.

Wasting time or not realizing how important it is to take advantage of your time used for a certain period in an activity that you can earn money or rewarded money trading your time.

In the old world or in history sometimes the trade for time was some type of commodity. For example, when men worked the field for farmers, in return farmers gave the men food, place to sleep, cloths or paid for medical needs and medication. That was the days when "time was precious" and now that precious turn to money, such as Gold, Silver, and Diamond. Managing Editor Eddie Adel

TRAVEL, FAVORITE PLACES CONNECTIONS AND HANGOUTS

LOOKING FOR LUXURY BREAK IDEAS IN FRANCE? *by Nathan Hicks*

If you are looking for a luxury break away in France, then why not consider chateau accommodation instead of a run-of-the-mill hotel? Costs are not as dramatic as the architecture appears.

When people think of a luxury break in France, almost always the very first thing to consider is staying in a luxury chateau. But how many people actually know what a chateau is? A chateau is a French word for a manor house or country estate home, similar to an English mansion, or stately home, originally housing a lord and/or lady of the manor. Chateaux have come to symbolize elegant extravagance and an aesthetically pleasing architecture, almost reminiscent of the pure embodiment of a childhood fairy tale castle, mansion house or stately home. Chateau accommodation in France is therefore the epitome of luxury when considering a break.

Chateaux date back to as far as the tenth century in France and so share many historical traits with other architectural buildings of interest from the same era. Usually built and framed within large parkland interspersed by interesting and ornate trees and finely sketched out gardens, chateaux lend themselves to grandeur and a certain €je ne sais quoi€. It is often this mystery appeal that brings people to the Northern France region of Normandy where there are many chateaux to choose from when considering chateau accommodation in France.

So, have you always wanted to visit France and get an authentic French experience? Want to witness first-hand the luxury accommodations and relaxing environment enjoyed by the other half? Want a plush and safe environment in which to lay your head after sightseeing, fit for a lord or lady? Many chateau accommodations in France are close to many sightseeing destinations, aside from the chateau itself. Different rooms and a vast array of suites are available to choose from. Beautiful views right from your very own chateau. Most chateaux are situated close to markets and restaurants for you to enjoy your local stay. France of course is also renowned for its wide and famous varieties of local wines, cheeses, meats and fruits. Tasting days are also popular activities typically, in the nearby vicinities. Museums also abound in Normandy, to pique the interest of any discerning visitor.

There are literally dozens of chateaux in the region of Normandy. So whether you are looking for a plush place to stay in Lower or Upper Normandy, whether it be in Calvados, Manche, Oren, Eure or Seine-Maritime, there is quite literally a place for everyone's style and taste. Perhaps you want to be near to the coastline. Perhaps you want to be tucked away in the stunning French countryside. Whatever the case, searching for a chateau accommodation in France is a simple and pleasurable experience when you search online.

So if you desire to see the Bayeux Tapestry and other medieval sites such as the Mont Saint Michel island, then booking chateau accommodation in France may be just the thing for you. Perhaps you want to experience history first-hand and follow in the footsteps of William the Conqueror or visit the World War II memorials at Normandy beach there is no finer way to travel and stay in chateau accommodation in France.

7 MOST SAFE CITIES ON THE PLANET EARTH IN 2015

Related factors are personal safety , crimes, accidents, and arrests. Health, major terminal illness and disease. Environment and the quality of air/ water, and pollution.. Cyber security, Identity theft, digital safety, privacy, and security from identity theft. Infrastructure, road safety, freeway safety, roads, building, and transportation safety. Tokyo took first place, , followed by Singapore, Osaka japan, Stockholm, Amsterdam, Sidney, and Zurich.

This was a study by EU using 50 cities around the world from LA, to NYC which came in the number ten spot, Toronto Canada, and the rest of Europe, Asia, Africa, and the Middle East.

Also among the cities in the study are: Hong Kong, San Francisco, Taipei, Montreal, Barcelona, Chicago, London, Washington, Frankfurt, Madrid, Br ussels, Paris, Seoul, Abu Dhabi, Milan, Rome, Santiago, Doha, Shanghai, Buenos Aires, Shenzhen, Lima, Tianjin, Rio de Janeiro, Kuwait City, Beijing, Guangzhou, Bangkok, Sao Paulo, Istanbul, Delhi, Moscow, M umbai, Mexico City, Riyadh, Johannesburg, Ho Chi Minh City, Tehran and Jakarta.

Study By EU, publish by The Daily Mail, UK.

Shopping • Fashion

FASHION, YOU AND I

• By Ajay Sharma •

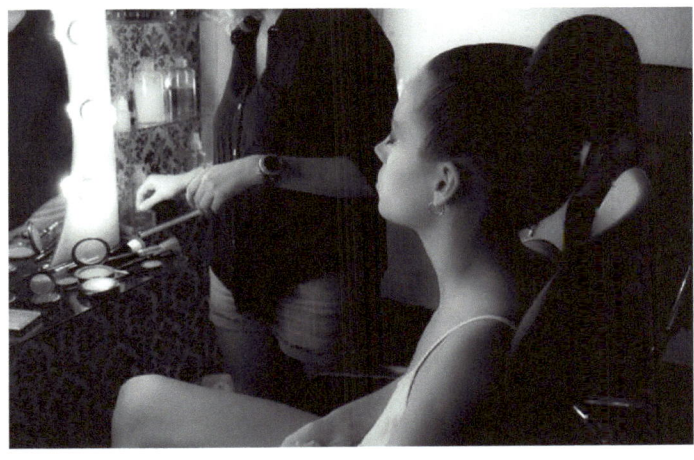

The thing about fashion is that it's ubiquitous. Whether it's your worn-out pair of sneakers or your ripped boyfriend jeans or your chic leather jacket, you are fashion, and fashion is you. Whatever be your personal style, fashion's got a name for it. Every item of clothing, footwear and accessories in your wardrobe is the heart and soul of fashion. That's the thing —fashion isn't all about the glitz and glam, it's just who you are, and how you choose to show it.

So you see? As much as people tend to think of fashion as something that's only for all the skinny girls of the world —they're wrong, it's for you and me, for everybody. Fashion isn't about being the perfect Size 0, or even a voluptuous hourglass oozing confidence and free-spiritedness, fashion is everything, fashions life!

So whether you've done an extensive course from a **fashion university** and picked up all the inner workings of the fashion industry, or whether you're just the girl next door with a closet full of plain tees and denim, fashion is A and Z, and everything in between. And when I speak for myself, I'm not the biggest fashion buff, but I've come to realize that fashion is in the air we breathe. Fashion is in your tastes, your likes and your dislikes, your look and your personal style.

Whether you're a graduate from the fashion institute of technology or whether you're a lawyer or a dancer or a cook or a writer, fashion is in you as much as it is in all those glossy cover page photos of the best fashion magazines. You don't need to keep up with the trends, or know all the secrets of a fashion university degree to have your own personal style. You don't need the latest shape of sunglasses to define your own fashion, you create who you are, and fashion is a little part of that —whether you like to admit it or not.

Of course, a degree in fashion is just going to help you understand yourself —and the world- better, but who says you need a certificate from the fashion institute of technology, or some such institute, to claim your own in the world of fashion? That's just it —the world of fashion isn't exclusively for all the models and designers of the world, you and I are just as much a part of it.

ABOUT THE AUTHOR

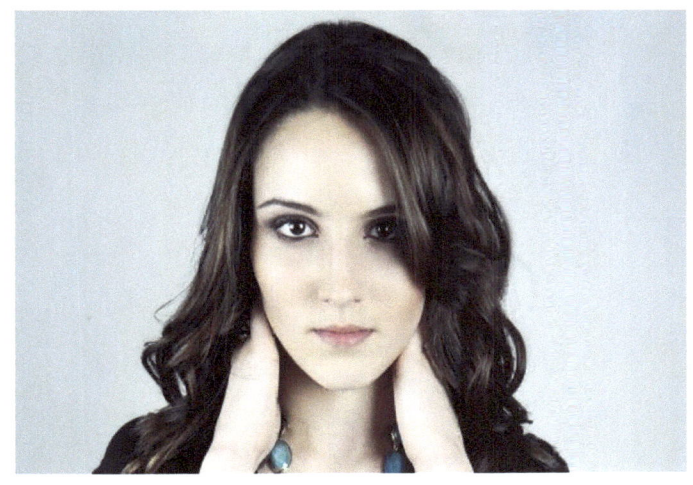

Ajay Sharma jay Sharma is professional content writer and publisher. He writes for his personal blogs, websites and for many content publishing...

CELEBRATE IN FASHION BY SPORTING MOTHER OF THE BRIDE DRESSES 2015

• By ramseomaster •

A daughter's wedding is the most emotional and poignant moment for a mother. You simply can't get away by looking drab on that day. Celebrate and cherish the moment with a stunning, elegant dress, complimenting the bride's outfit, for it will create that perfect picture memoir, helping you recall the special day.

You should wear something which is sober, graceful and in some lighter shades like **Silver Mother of the Bride Dresses** or darker ones, but not bright colors as it is a distraction and puts off people. Don't be anxious or nervous about carrying it off as you will get a lot of options regarding the sizes. Slim, curvy or plus sized, the online portals take care of all your needs. Choose the dresses which will highlight your best features and hide the flabby body parts. Dark colored, nicely fitted dresses help you look slimmer. You can visit www.ericdress.com/ for a quick reference of **2015 mother of the bride dresses**.

You will get a variety of choices regarding the shapes, color, style, fabric, sleeves, etc. A-lines, columns, mermaids etc. are some popular silhouettes on offer. Traditional mother of the bride dresses are floor length and mostly come in natural waistlines although empire ones are also available. Zippers make the **mother of the bride dresses 2015** easy to wear while some bold mommas may go for a backless gown. Some of the popular necklines are V-necks, off the shoulders, sweetheart, jeweled etc. Most dresses have embellished beads and appliqués. For more glamour, select a dress with a train. Chiffon,

satin, velvet and lace are the chiefly fabrics for these dresses. Lighter shades of colors like peach, mauve, pink, gold, teal or dark blue and violet are extremely well-received. **Silver Mother of the Bride Dresses** is a time-tested, safe and traditional option.

You can select the dress according to the type of wedding event as well, like receptions, parties or the marriage itself. Keep accessories and make-up to the minimum. Select properly fitted shoes. These will help you take confident and graceful strides as quite expectantly, you would be a busy bee on the D-day. Also, keep the budget in mind. There are a lot of sites likewww.ericdress.com/list/cheap-mother-of-the-bride-dresses-2015-105207/ which offer cheap **2015 mother of the bride dresses** and that too, at a discounted price.

Select your favored color and size from the drop down menu carefully while ordering **mother of the bride dresses 2015**. Don't forget to get your beloved daughter's advice.

So go ahead. Buy the perfect dress and create a beautiful memory.

By:

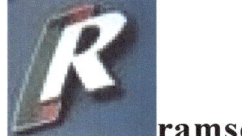 **ramseomaster**

Ericdress is the best place that you can find for the dresses for the bride and for her mother. Once you visit us you won't be disappointed...

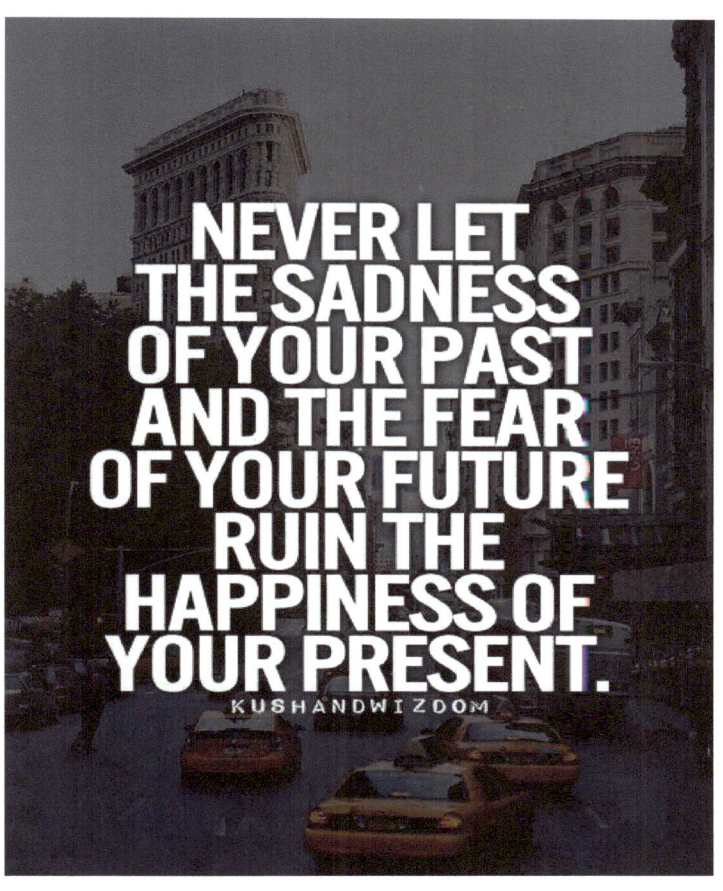

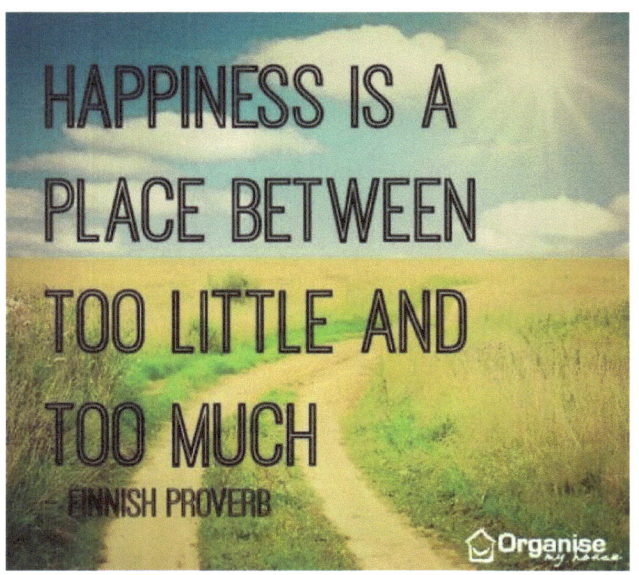

THERE ARE
SO MANY
BEAUTIFUL
REASONS
TO BE
HAPPY

A SECRET TO
HAPPINESS IS LETTING
EVERY SITUATION BE
WHAT IT IS, INSTEAD
OF WHAT YOU THINK
IT SHOULD BE.
LOUBIS - AND - CHAMPAGNE

BASIC HEALTH AND SAFETY IN THE WORKPLACE

May 13, 2015 • By Samara Weidmann •

Before 1956 there weren't any laws that affected Health and Safety, but come along "The Agriculture Health and Safety act", ultimately this was developed to ensure all workers and even children were kept safe around agricultural apparatus. Out of all the laws, the most important one must have been the investigation and reporting of disease or accidents (which still today plays a big part in society!)

Come 1974, a revolutionary act was created which changed Healthy and Safety in the workplace for everyone, it was called "The Health and Safety at Work act" and when this was introduced it was meant to connect with both employers and employees. To ensure that this act was forced and regulated, the HSC (the Health and Safety Commission) was founded. Along come the eighties, 1981 was when the HSC decided it was time to introduce the Health and Safety First Aid regulations, this demanded that an employer must ensure the appropriate first aid equipment is available to all workers.

With there being so many different workplace hazards, such as chemicals, electricity, heat sources, machinery, manual handling and even slip and trip hazards just to name a few... you can really see why these regulations have become a requirement for all workplaces to follow and why having the appropriate equipment is a must for all employees!

What is appropriate equipment? Ultimately it depends on what your job role includes, for example: A builder:

Head protection (hard hat) would protect them against head impact. **Eye protection** (goggles) to ensure that wind or air movement won't blow dust or particles into their eyes.

Hand protection (gloves) ultimately this will protect them from cuts, slivers, punctures or even electricity.

Foot protection (boots) they need them to protect them from the impact of falling or rolling objects, slippery or uneven surfaces, stepping on sharp objects and even electrical hazards.

Hearing protection (ear defenders) if they are working in a noisy environment, they will require these to protect them from excessive noise.

High visibility clothing (high vies vest) should the workers be working at night, or in low light, they should wear one.

Breathing protection (dust mask) in some scenarios, the builder may be working around potentially dangerous vapors or even just dust could be dangerous.

Here I have found a website which provides some fantastic work wear for all your safety needs, at great prices: http://jcbworkwear.com/uk/

Hope this is has helped!

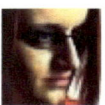

SAMARA WEIDMANN

Hi my name is Samara Weidmann. I am regarded as an expert when it comes to health and safety in the workplace, having helped numerous companies improves their own health and safety procedures. If you are looking for tips and information on work safety wear or require advice on the importance of safety at work including PPE (Personal Protective Equipment), then my articles will certainly help you. In my spare time, I enjoy activities that get the adrenaline pumping, such as bungee jumping, rock climbing and abseiling down cliff sides.

HOW TO HANDLE HOT BEVERAGE, COFFEE IN A PAPER CUP TO GO

May 14, 2015 • By Eddie Elchahed •

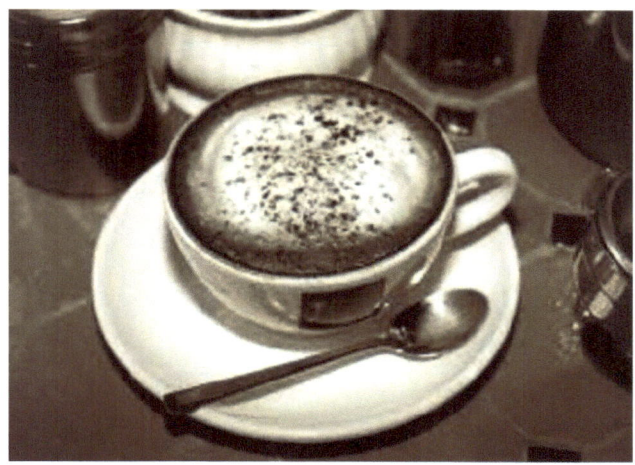

I can say that today handeling food like any other career full of regulations. Health and safety rules for everything, employment regulations for fairness among employees, labor laws, and food and beverage temerature.

Recently, Starbucks Coffee Company in Ralligh North Carolina was found ""not liable for damages" for a cop who filed a lawsuit against the coffee maker for spilling his coffee cup in his lap and received third degree burns three years ago. The leutenant law suit asking for $750,000. Damages for the incident that caused him severe stress, triggering his crohn's disease and leading to surgery to remove part of his intestine.

The story was published on 05/13/2015 in the Washington Post, and in the finding the officer was resposible for not seeking treatment immediately, he waited over two hours before he went to the doctor. If The coffee was extremely hot and caused third degree burns, the Leutenant should have gone to the Er immediately.

Hot coffee should never be placed in one lap. It doesn't matter how hot it is. Realizing that it is hot coffee is good enough reason.

The Leutenant claim that the lid puped out of the coffee cup causing spill in his lap. Lid do not just pup up for no reason. I myself a religious coffee drinker. i drink starbucks coffee all day, about six venty cups of starbucks coffee per day minimum, and never a lid just puped up by itself. Try it at home, with extra cautious. Do not place any hot liquid in your lap or someone else's lap. Just place the hot coffee cup on a table and wait, use common sense, couple of hours is enough for the lid to pup up. it will never happen.

I'am sure we all feel for the Leutenant and his personal injuries. My God he is only human. We support the fact that he was working on duty when it happened, and he is to receive all company medical care available, and all necessary treatments.

Starbucks coffee is at first hot at 200 degree, and this is what is best about it. We like starbucks coffee for the hot long lasting taste of the coffee and the osmosis filtered style water. The Starbucks cofffee is rotated all the time for best brewed taste, unless it ismy favorite and the company signature brand "Pike Place".
Eddie elchahed, Expert on Food and beverage

you can read more of my articles at weconnect2.com digital network.

ABOUT THE AUTHOR

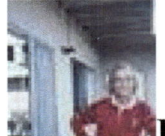 **Eddie Elchahed**

Eddie elchahed MBA in Marketing Management from National University Irvine Campus, Bachelor in Arts from CSUF in International Business...
Managing Editor, My Connections Magazine.

Food and Beverage • Restaurant Reviews

RESTAURANT STAFF

BEHAVIORS TIPS
• By Eddie Elchahed •

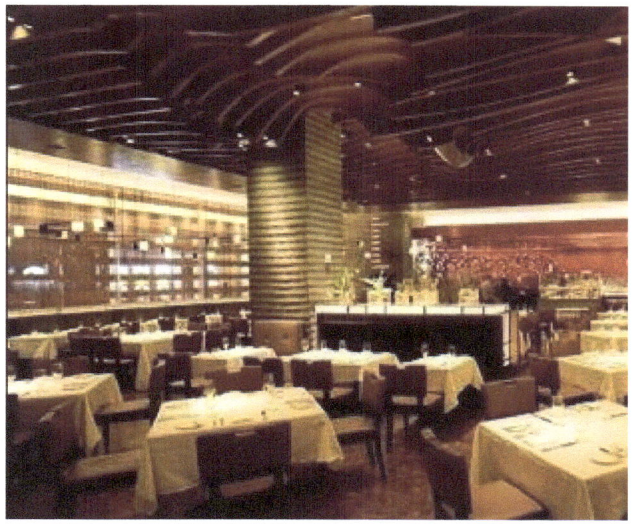

Restaurant continue to be an American Tradition. In every family around the nation someone is involve in a restaurant activity beside the customer part. Mom, dad, sister, brother, cousin, boyfriend, girlfriend, and on with the list is part of a restaurant operation. Sure sometimes more than one member of the family, or sometimes is all the family who become involved in the restaurant as a family business. For a long time , many restaurateurs have tried to minimize this people business to less and less people involved in the hands on operation. Today it become the front runner issue as labor cost climb and continue to rise above all other cost. The minimum wage in most state is about $15.00 per hour, and the spread nation wide is near the future.

Staff make the restaurant or break it. Although many restaurant companies top management tried to divert the idea to look as if they have stores to manage instead of people, few have made the stores management successful. It only last so far. This far as today and we can't guarantee the future of this so far short time success.

In brief, managing restaurants as STORES, is concern and focus more on the restaurant building inside out, including all the restaurant equipments, food and beverage products, dry good items, and to make this sort of short, let's say everything inside and outside the restaurant have higher priorities than the staffing. That the staff of the restaurant come and go, but the restaurant and what is invested in it will stay.

On the other hand, staffing is part of the people business, and this restaurant business is all about people. Staff are people too, and they are the heart and soul of the customers base.

Human resources it is called in many restaurant operations, and this part have special department to deal with. Labor laws, employment regulations, civil rights, safety, health issues, and staff development are part of this H&R Department. People are different in every way you try to imagine, and that what make the restaurant staffing a challenge.

How to put a team together that will cause the minimum amount of problems and continue to operate in good standing for making customers happy, and staying at least above standards for all major reports which signal positive results for everyday operation.

Staffing behavior for the most part take the majority of time from the management. Determine and decisive management at all level, make the decision of team work assignments based on their best knowledge of the staff over all abilities. Decisions filtering from top management to middle management, and down to operation management are extremely crucial to the everyday restaurant operation activities. To have choices is some other times when it is time to make every customer happy. Staff choices as who can be a shift leader, or who can be my manager, and who i can work with and can not, to jeopardize everything else so one or two staff can make their own choice which make them the only happy people around. Decisions effect behaviors of restaurant staff, and thus make the difference on customers satisfaction. Deciding how many people should work a shift, and who should make the team on that shift, it is steering the restaurant in the right direction. Staffing behaviors can be molded to positive and profitable depend on the decisions made by management toward the staff from

training, feedback, teamwork, and
rewarding and reminding.

FUNNY PHOTO

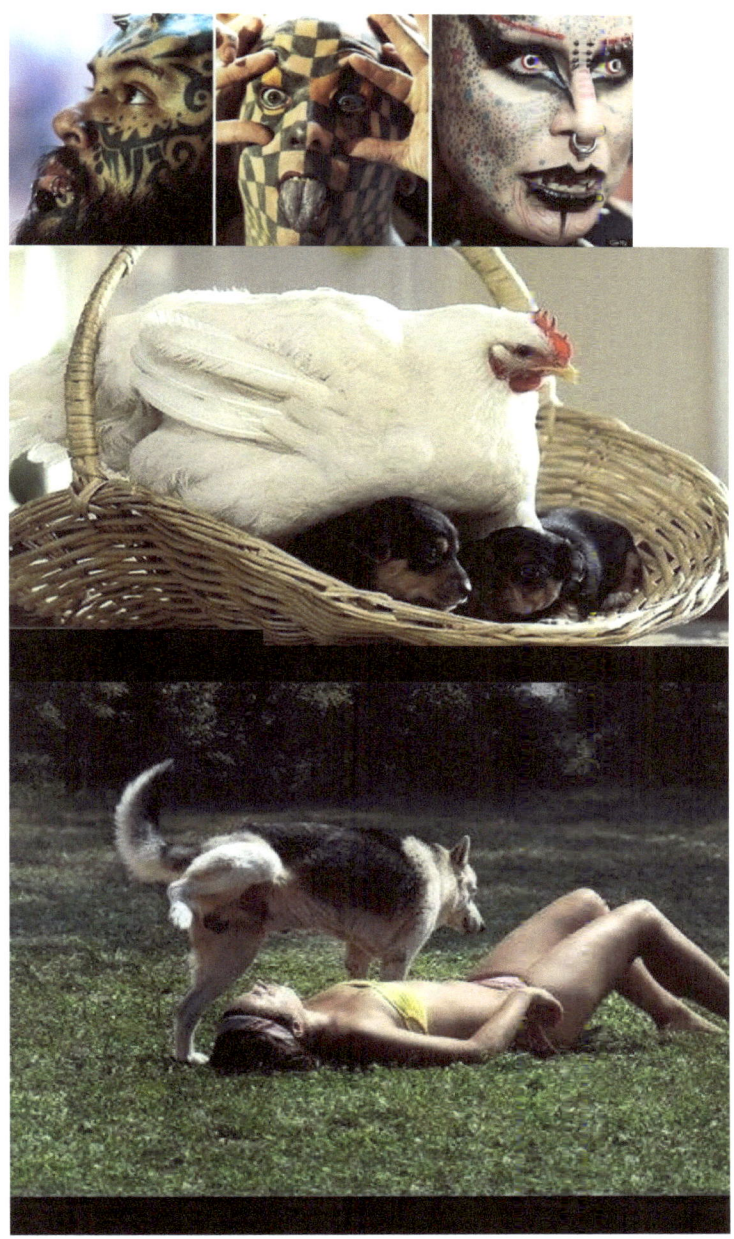

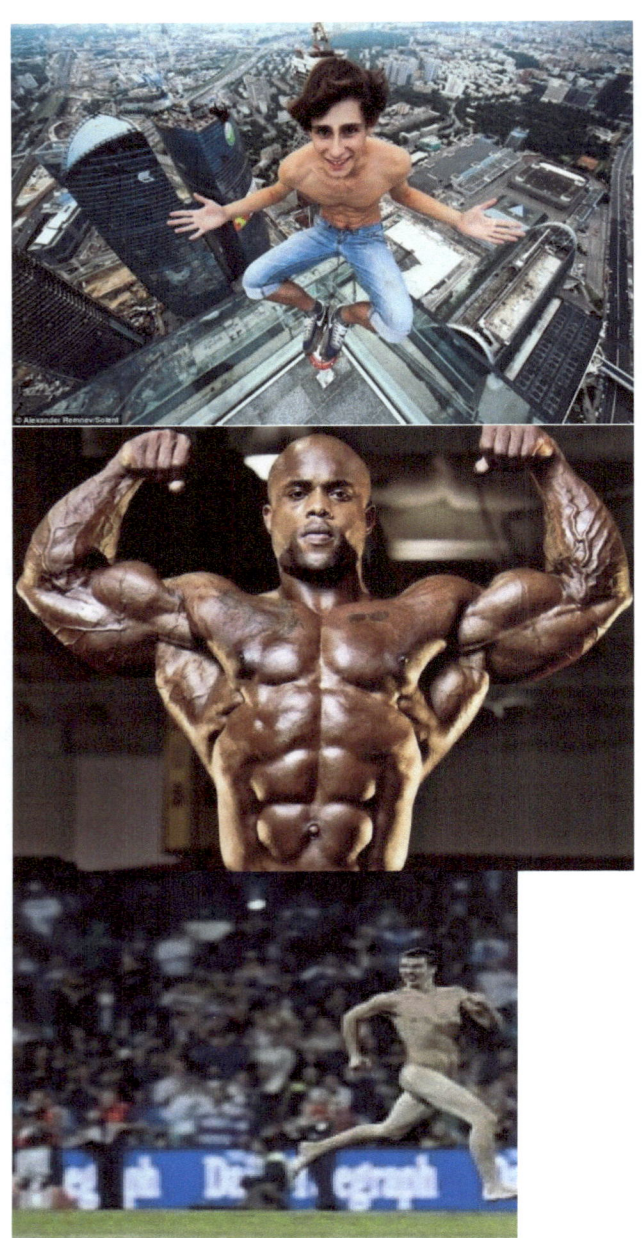

AMAZING PLACES, CAVES, AND
WORLD WONDERS PYRAMIDS.

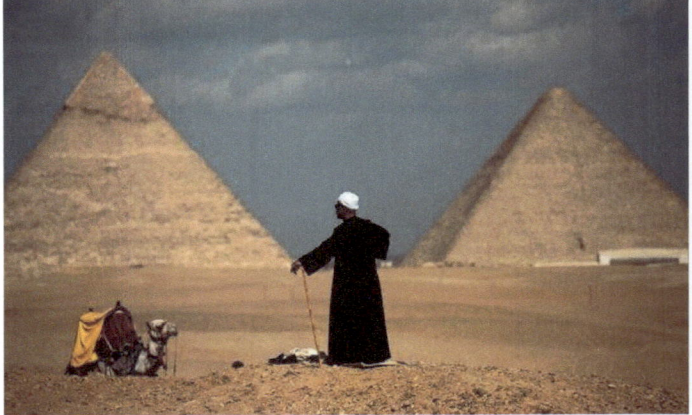

A camel driver waits for tourists near the Pyramids at Giza.

Tourism is Egypt's second largest source of revenue, bringing in $13 billion in 2010. The Great Pyramid at Giza, after all, is one of the seven ancient wonders of the world.

Who Built them?

The question of who labored to build them, and why, has long been part of their fascination. Rooted firmly in the popular imagination is the idea that the pyramids were built by slaves serving a merciless pharaoh. This notion of a vast slave class in Egypt originated in Judeo-Christian tradition and has been popularized by Hollywood productions like Cecil B. De

Mille's *The Ten Commandments*, in which a captive people labor in the scorching sun beneath the whips of pharaoh's overseers. But graffiti from inside the Giza monuments themselves have long suggested something very different.

Until recently, however, the fabulous art and gold treasures of pharaohs like Tutankhamen have overshadowed the efforts of scientific archaeologists to understand how human forces—perhaps all levels of Egyptian society—were mobilized to enable the construction of the pyramids. Now, drawing on diverse strands of evidence, from geological history to analysis of living arrangements, bread-making technology, and animal remains, Egyptologist Mark Lehner, an associate of Harvard's Semitic Museum, is beginning to fashion an answer. He has found the city of the pyramid builders. They were not slaves.

CRYSTAL CAVE

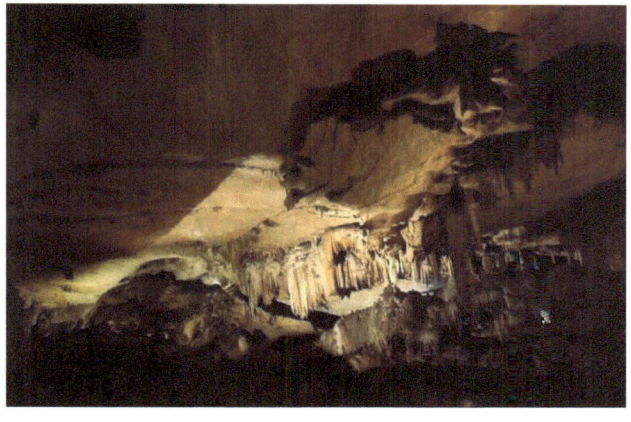

Sequoia National Park, in the U.S. state of California is home of 240 known caves. Crystal Cave is a marble cave which is park's second-longest at over 3.4 miles. It is in the Giant Forest region, between the Ash Mountain entrance of the park and Giant Forest. The cave is a constant 9 °C (48 °F), and only accessible by guided tour.

Education • College and University

ORIGINS OF BEHAVIOR AND THE SOCIAL LEARNING THEORY

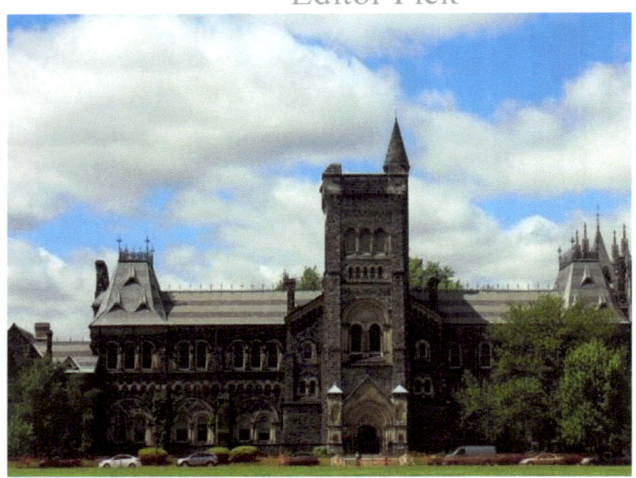

Origins of behaviors have over the years remained controversial and of great interest among different groups of people. This is in relation to all living organisms ranging from human beings to ants. Research on the field of behaviors has shown that each group of population behave arbitrary distinctive in reference to a binary choice of problem (Junginger, Claypoole & Renilo-Laygo, 2006). It has also been realized that offspring of the initial population behave identically to their parents. Junginger, Claypoole & Renilo-Laygo (2006) indicated that that behaviors linked to reproductive success will always survive while those that are less reproductively successful will disappear at exponential rates. Different theories have been established concerning origins of behaviors. In this regards, social learning theory has been the most outstanding, whereby it has explicitly demonstrated the concept of origins of behaviors.

Social learning theory was proposed by Albert Bandura, whereby it is rooted to the basic concepts of traditional learning theory. The theory postulates that people can learn new behaviors and information through watching other people (Rotter, 2000). The main issue focused by this theory is the role of observations in modeling human behavior. The idea of internal mental states has also been identified to be influential in demonstration and development of human behavior. Nevertheless, the theory has gone further to state that learning does not primarily lead to a change in behavior. As outlined by Rotter (2000), the key steps involved in modeling process and observational learning include; attention, retention, reproduction, and motivation. All the steps are integrated and equally important in the learning process, thus leading to establishment of new behaviors.

The ideas and insights propagated by the social learning theory are of great importance in human life. This is basically in the influencing of positive or socially acceptable behaviors (Bartol & Bartol, 2011). People are able to observe and learn admirable behaviors of other people within their communities, thus able to lead better life. For instance, the youth can adequately adopt the insights of this theory to imitate the behaviors of heroes in their society. This is achieved through close attention, retention, reproduction,
and motivation to imitate the behaviors (Bartol & Bartol, 2011). As a result of this phenomenon, desirable values and behaviors are able to grow across all members of the society.

Self Improvement • Psychology

CHANGING BEHAVIORS USING PSYCHOLOG

• BY **HELPING PSYCHOLOGY** •

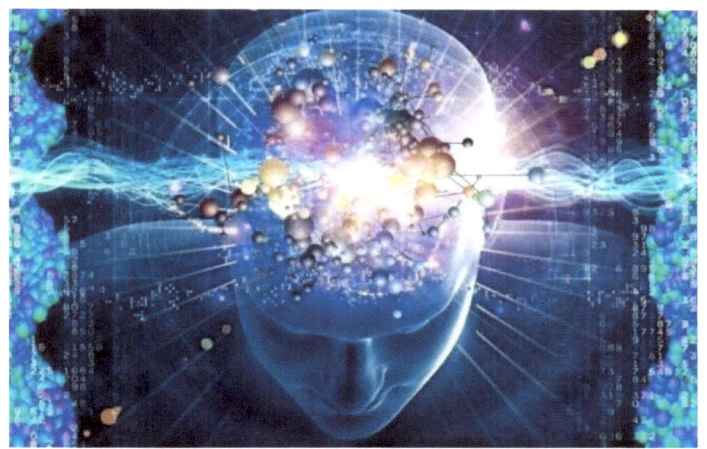

Making a lasting behavioral change is not an easy task. It is a challenge that requires a strong commitment of time and effort. One of the main **steps to changing a behavior is to set goals**. This includes monitoring progress in achieving those goals and making adjustments as needed. The keys to success are persistence and motivation.

Psychologists have developed several ways to help people change their behavior in order to improve their quality of life. Three of the most effective methods are as follows:

1) Stages of Change

"5 stages of change" was first introduced in the late 1970s by researchers James Prochaska and Carlo DiClemente while researching ways to quit smoking. Change occurs gradually. In the early stages, there is often an unwillingness or resistance to change. But as time passes, people develop a commitment to the new behavior. This method is effective in weight loss, to quit smoking and to improve study habits.

Three important elements in "stages of change" are readiness to change, barriers to change and expecting relapses. Readiness to change simply means that the person must be willing to use the knowledge and resources necessary to make a lasting change. A person should identify the barriers to change and take steps to avoid them. Occasional relapses are expected, but only recognized as minor setbacks. Lasting success depends on reaffirming goals and persistence.

2) Operant Conditioning

"Operant conditioning," also known as instrumental conditioning, was introduced by a behaviorist, **B. F. Skinner**, while studying the association between a behavior and its consequences. This method of behavioral change uses the elements of reward and punishment as a motivator to change. The promise of a reward generates a positive reinforcement for a particular behavior. On the contrary, the promise of punishment generates a negative reinforcement.

An example of "operant conditioning" may be used for employees. Hard working employees are rewarded for their good work ethic with pay raises or promotions; hard work is reinforced and encouraged. On the other hand, slothful employees are punished by reprimand, pay cuts or demotions; laziness is decreased and discouraged. This method of behavioral change is also very effective in child discipline. Good behavior is rewarded with praise; bad behavior is decreased by scolding.

3) Classical Conditioning

"Classical conditioning" was discovered by **Ivan Pavlov, a Russian physiologist**. This method uses the associations between an environmental stimulus and a naturally occurring stimulus to change behaviors. Classical conditioning is useful in the treatment of phobias or anxiety problems. By pairing an anxiety provoking situation with pleasant surroundings, this helps people change their behavior through new associations. Feelings of fear and anxiety are replaced with relaxation.

To treat a person who has a fear of speaking in front of others, a technique called "systematic desensitization," is very effective. The person is given various opportunities to speak in front of a group, either in role playing or reality situations, with the addition of calming techniques. Eventually, the person learns to relax in front of a group. Fear is replaced by relaxation so that the fear of public speaking is eliminated all together.

For patients in need of a behavioral change, the most effective treatments involve listening, understanding and slow progression to ensure lasting results.

Helping Psychology

Helping Psychology is your guide to learning more about the Psychology profession and the opportunities that are available in this dynamic..

_____

_____

Business • Training

DIFFERENTIAL REINFORCEMENT IS A PREFERRED METHOD TO BEHAVIOR CHANGE PROGRAMS WITH DOGS THAN USING PUNISHMENT

• By Niki Tudge •

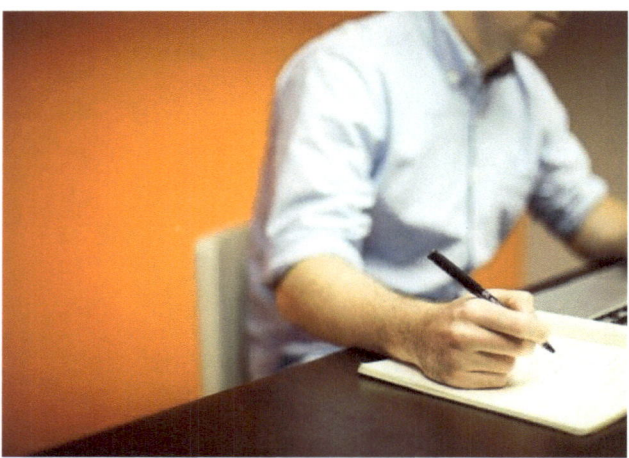

Punishment has sinister and subtle side effects, it drives problem behaviors underground and they tend to then be displayed in the absence of the punisher. Punishment also activates the dogs' emotional system which has a negative impact on the dogs' ability to think and learn making it almost impossible to teach the dog new more acceptable behaviors.

Because punishment can never be applied consistently and predictability this leads to learned helplessness, a state resistant to rehabilitation, as the dog cannot control nor have confidence in its environment (O'Heare 2004).

A successful behavior change program must make the problematic target behavior ineffective, irrelevant and inefficient. The program must also establish new behaviors and skills while decreasing the frequency, intensity or duration of problem behaviors. Since punishment can create many problems, alternative methods of modifying unwanted behavior, such as differential reinforcement, are preferable (Miltenberger 2004)

Differential reinforcement is an operant conditioning technique that can be used to both increase and decrease behaviors. For many problematic operant behaviors during differential reinforcement, the problematic behavior is targeted for extinction while another behavior is simultaneously positively reinforced. There are several differential reinforcement protocols and each has its application and suitability based on the behavioral problem.

When choosing a differential reinforcement protocol we must first establish whether the target behavior is already present and requires a dimension of the behavior to be reduced, such as barking, or whether the goal is to place the old behavior on extinction and reinforce a new behavior, such as jumping on guests when sitting would be more acceptable.

When considering which differential reinforcement protocol to use for teaching new behaviors we need to assess if the preferred behavior is already occurring, can it be captured or lured or will it need to be shaped. We also need to establish if we will use extinction trials or not and whether given the behavior problem they may create frustration or cause

an animal to aggress, both causing frustration during training or a trigger of aggression are considered training failures and should be avoided at all costs (O'Heare 2009).

Differential Reinforcement of an incompatible behavior is best used when we can identify an incompatible behavior, a behavior that is physically incompatible with the problem behavior and one that commonly occurs so it can be captured or prompted easily without exposing the animal to the problem stimulus. We must have access to a reinforcer that can be delivered after the new behavior and the ability to withhold reinforcement for the undesirable behavior.

The new incompatible behavior is trained in a different context to the problem behavior and then exposed gradually to the problem stimulus to avoid extinction trials as this can result in aggression and extinction bursts. If a dog is jumping all over people as they come in through a door we would first teach a solid sit for greetings away from the door and then gradually move the behavior back to the problem location. If an incompatible behavior cannot be identified then, using the same methods, we can differentially reinforce a specific alternate behavior (O'Heare 2009).

When working with an animal that is highly excitable or has a propensity to engage in frustration behaviors, such as nipping or mouthing, then one should adopt the differential reinforcement protocol of "other behavior". This is a simple procedure where the reinforcer is contingent on the absence of the problem behavior. Reinforcement is easily accessed by the animal and the procedure is easily carried out by the owner. Because there is no specifically targeted behavior to reinforce the technician must remain cognizant that differential reinforcement of other behaviors can create superstitious behaviors (O'Heare 2009).

With behavior that cannot be reduced to zero (barking) or some level of the behavior is acceptable and/or it is difficult to train an incompatible or alternate behavior, then using differential reinforcement of low rates is used. It would first be determined whether the goal of the behavior change program is to reduce the intensity, frequency or duration of the baking behavior and the protocol would then focus on that behavior dimension. Reinforcement would then only be available to the animal if the specific target behavior occurred at a specified rate during a specified period of time (O'Heare 2009).

If the goal of the behavior change program is to establish a new replacement behavior and the animal being trained lacks social confidence or offers ridged behaviors as a result of previously harsh or aversive training protocols then using differential reinforcement of successive approximations to a terminal behavior (shaping) would be most appropriate.

Shaping can also be used to develop operant behaviors that are not initially visible, need to be trained in small approximations or the conditions of the training need to support empowering the animal to experiment with new behaviors. Shaping procedures can also be used to teach alternative or incompatible behaviors without the use of extinction trials. A key benefit to using shaping and differential reinforcement protocols is that they also positively impact the animal's respondent behavior (O'Heare 2009).

Differential reinforcement protocols that focus on operant extinction are designed to decrease behaviors by withholding or preventing any reinforcement for the problem behavior. If it is necessary to use protocols that focus on extinction trials because other less invasive or aversive methods have been tried and failed the extinction procedures should always be used with a reinforcement procedure of a desirable behavior

Operant extinction trials for aggressive behavior should only be used when the behavior is positively reinforced, i.e. the positive reinforcer is no longer delivered after the behavior, most aggression behaviors are negatively reinforced, and the dog exhibits the behavior to remove the stimulus from its environment.

Miltenberger (2004) Behavior Modification Principles and Procedures Third Edition, Thompson. USA

O'Heare, J. (2008) Behavior Change Programming and Procedures 2009, CASI Course Notes,

O'Heare, J. (2004) Canine Separation Anxiety Workbook 5th Edition DogPsych Publishing Canada

Niki Tudge is the owner and founder of The DogSmith, America's Dog Training, Dog Walking and Pet Care Franchise. CPDT, E-Nadoi, CBC,AABP-..

_____

_____

Negative Behaviors at work…..

NEGATIVE THOUGHTS AND TALK CAN HURT YOUR COMPANY

• By Patricia Woloch •

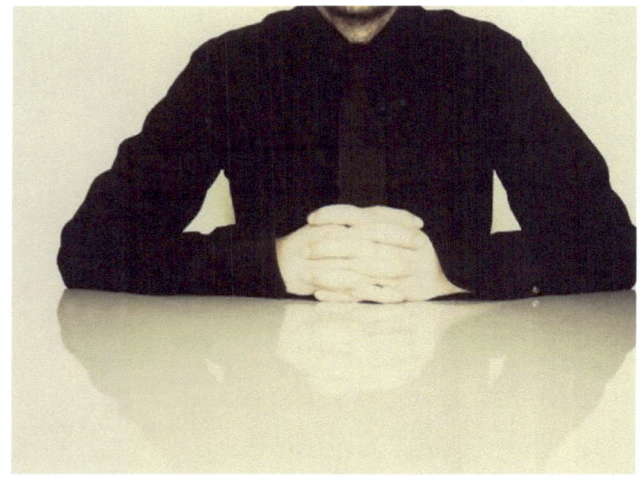

At some time or another, organizations and businesses may struggle with employees' negative attitudes. Often, these shifts in attitude can be linked to organization trauma such asdownsizing, budget cuts or workload increases, but sometimes negative attitudes evolve with no apparent triggers. Increased complaining, a focus on why things aren't getting done, and a lack of hope that things will get better may characterize negative employees' behavior. Staff negativity can make your whole company feel as though it's in a rut, and negativity is certainly contagious. Negativism can even affect the most positive employees.

There are ways, however, that managers can deal with negative employee behavior and thinking including:

1. Model positive behavior. If management is acting and talking negatively, staff will certainly follow; managers must model positive

company behavior. Additionally, take a positive approach by showing confidence in your employees' abilities. Expect a lot from your staff, support them in their efforts, hold them accountable, and be clear in your expectations. Good managers will set standards for their own work and employee relations and meet those standards, setting an example of positive behavior.

2. Acknowledge existing negativity. Ignoring negativity will not make it go away. If you don't acknowledge the negativity, then your employees may view you as being out of touch and not aware of your company's dynamic. Acknowledge the negativity your perceive, and do not try to convince your employees that they shouldn't have those negative feelings. Instead, ask for suggestions regarding what to do about the negativity and come up with solutions together.

3. Identify the positives. Look for small victories and discuss them. Turning a negative company into a positive one is the result of many little actions.

4. Provide positive reinforcement and recognition often. Provide positive recognition as soon as you find out about good performance, and do not couple positive strokes with suggestions for improvement. Those two things must be separated as combining them devalues the recognition.

5. Don't ever go along with the negativity. Regardless of your position in the combination, it can be easy sometimes to participate in the negative talk that is taking place around the water cooler. When faced with negative conversations, consider changing the subject, comment on the negative content ("Hey, let's move on to something more pleasant."), or ask what can be done to remedy the

situation that is causing negative feelings.

One of the age-old questions in the sales world is "Are leaders born or made?" Regardless of which school of thought you subscribe to, gifted sales managers often attain their position by demonstrating competence in the sales arena and modeling good sales and good company behavior. High-performing sales organizations apply the best practices, and perceiving, acknowledging and addressing negative employee behavior and attitude is crucial to ensuring success for you and your company.

POLICING THE COMMUNITIES HAS CHANGED.

THE SIMPLE STRATEGIES THAT COULD FUNDAMENTALLY CHANGE HOW COMMUNITIES VIEW THEIR POLICE

The president, police experts, activists and even some police officers have called for major changes to the American law enforcement system. Community policing -- used in Columbia Heights, Minnesota, where Captain Lenny Austin is seen here mentoring a student in 2013 -- might just be the change police departments need. (Photo: Richard Sennott/Star Tribune/ZUMA Press/Corbis)

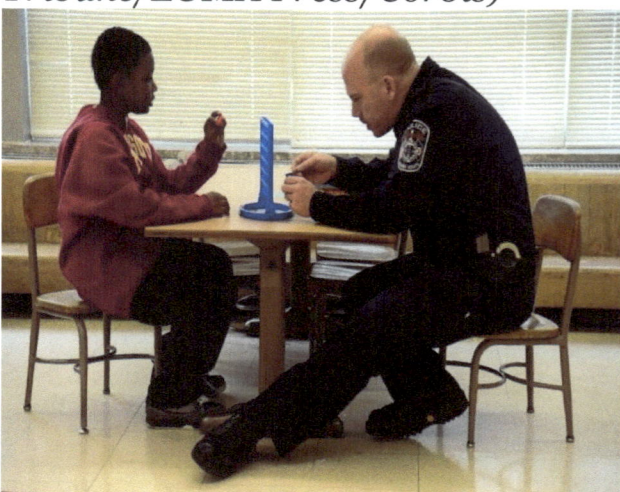

Raising a black son, Gail Howard couldn't shake the fear that someday, he was going to get shot. She even saw a therapist, who told her the odds were higher that she'd win the lottery. Jordan, an A student and an athlete, wanted her to relax, too -- he told her she treated him like a baby. The 17-year-old spent the entire day of Jan. 5, 2011, begging his mother for permission to walk alone to meet up with friends. Eventually, she grudgingly gave in.

"I said, 'We'll see how safe this town is once your eyes are looking down the barrel of a gun,'" Howard, who lives in Redlands, California, told The Huffington Post. "Those were the last words I spoke to him, and then 15 minutes later I get a phone call, he's shot in the eye."

Jordan and one of his friends were lucky enough to survive the gang shooting that took place that day; two other boys who were with them at the playground were not. Over the course of the yearlong investigation that followed, Howard -- who had previously had few interactions with police -- began to see local police officers as partners rather than patrolmen, forging bonds that would last far beyond the investigation and inspire her to begin fighting for the city's kids.

"They did not stop until they figured out who shot my boy and his friends," Howard said of the Redlands police, who eventually caught the shooters; they were convicted and sentenced to life behind bars. "I'm forever grateful to them."

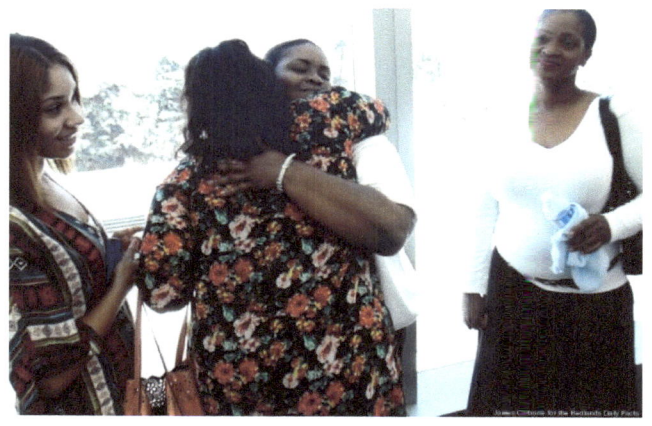

GAIL HOWARD, RIGHT, LOOKS ON AS A FELLOW MOTHER OF A VICTIM IN THE 2011 REDLANDS SHOOTING HUGS A RELATIVE, SHORTLY AFTER THREE MEN RECEIVED LIFE SENTENCES FOR THE CRIME. (PHOTO: *James Carbone* FOR THE *Redlands Daily Facts*)

Howard's attitude may come as a surprise at a time when relations between many police departments and their communities appear strained. The public remains outraged over the deaths of Michael Brown and Eric Garner and the subsequent failure to indict the police officers who killed them. In fact, there seems to be one thing nearly everyone agrees on after the months of protests those killings inspired: The relationships between American police and the communities they protect, particularly minority communities, are in need of serious repair.

"The system of policing has earned our mistrust," said Opal Tometi, a New York-based activist and co-founder of the #BlackLivesMatter campaign. In many ways, Tometi's group embodies the recent decline in relations between police and communities.

#BlackLivesMatter protests across the country have called for reformsincluding increased accountability surrounding police shootings and a reduction in the use of military equipment by local police departments. The shooting of two New York City police officers shortly after the announcement of the Garner verdict further intensified the national debate on policing in America. But beyond the headlines, many police forces are working to build trust with their communities. Police experts say that improved relations can be attributed largely to common-sense approaches that build on the philosophy known as community policing.

"Ordinary, good police work is not terribly newsworthy," said Gary Cordner, a professor of criminal justice at Kutztown University, "but lots and lots of good, ordinary police work goes on every day just about everywhere."

In the wake of recent police killings, national leaders and local police departments are increasingly turning to the community policing model that cities like Redlands have relied on for years. People like Gail and Jordan Howard are proof that the model can deliver on its promise of helping police and communities work together.

At a time of strained police relations, community-oriented policing offers a different approach -- one that makes good relationships essential to good police work.

The U.S. Department of Justice's Community Oriented Policing Services office defines community policing as "a philosophy that promotes organizational strategies, which support the systematic use of partnerships and problem-solving techniques, to proactively address the immediate conditions that give rise to public safety issues such as crime, social disorder and fear of crime."

Some police departments began emphasizing community policing during the 1970s, in response to the political unrest and widespread protests of the 1960s. The nation was reeling from incidents like the 1965 Watts Riots in Los Angeles, the protests that followed the assassination of Martin Luther King Jr. in 1968, the Stonewall Riots in 1969 and a number of anti-Vietnam War demonstrations that featured violent confrontations between police and civilians. The conditions were, as they are now, ripe for reform.

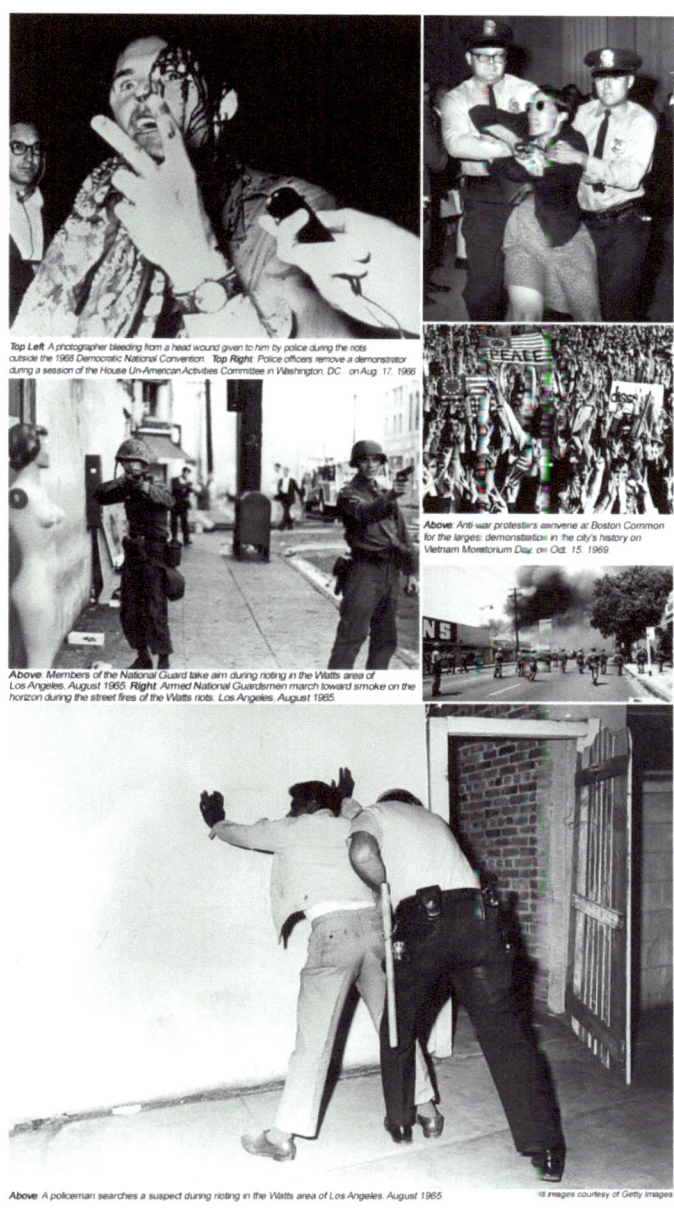

Top Left: A photographer bleeding from a head wound given to him by police during the riots outside the 1968 Democratic National Convention. Top Right: Police officers remove a demonstrator during a session of the House Un-American Activities Committee in Washington, DC. on Aug. 17, 1966

Above: Anti-war protesters convene at Boston Common for the largest demonstration in the city's history on Vietnam Moratorium Day, on Oct. 15, 1969

Above: Members of the National Guard take aim during rioting in the Watts area of Los Angeles, August 1965. Right: Armed National Guardsmen march toward smoke on the horizon during the street fires of the Watts riots. Los Angeles, August 1965.

Above: A policeman searches a suspect during rioting in the Watts area of Los Angeles, August 1965.   All images courtesy of Getty Images

In practice, community policing involves forming partnerships with community organizations, prioritizing transparency, actively pursuing feedback and establishing programs that allow police to engage with residents outside of the law enforcement arena. At its best, the practice allows community members to feel heard, respected and empowered to help police control crime in their neighborhoods, rather than feeling that officers are solely there to enforce laws through aggressive stopping, questioning, arresting and incarcerating.

"You can't arrest your way out of community problems," said Scott Nadeau, police chief of Columbia Heights, Minnesota. Nadeau took over the police department in 2008, and oversaw a shift to a community-focused approach. "That's something that I think is important for us as a community and us as a police agency to understand," he said. "Enforcement is a piece of the puzzle, but it's only one piece."

It's a strategy that seems simple, but it's far different from the way many departments operate.

Columbia Heights, an inner-ring Minneapolis suburb, was battling high

crime rates when Nadeau took over, bringing with him a background in community-oriented policing. Four years later, the department won aninternational award for community policing after crime hit a 25-year low. All officers in Nadeau's department are required to perform at least 10 hours of community policing activities every year, though he said most devote closer to 40 hours to the work. Officers are encouraged to choose activities that match their skills and interests. There are many choices: conducting CPR trainings, answering questions at classes for recent immigrants, serving food at a church's community dinner or holding "Coffee with a Cop" open hours, where residents are free to speak their minds with officers.

Nadeau said that community policing "wasn't always popular with [officers], it took months or years for some people to see the value." He noted that the department took care to introduce new initiatives slowly. "But I think even the officers we had that were more traditional saw the changes in the relationships between our police department and the community," he said.

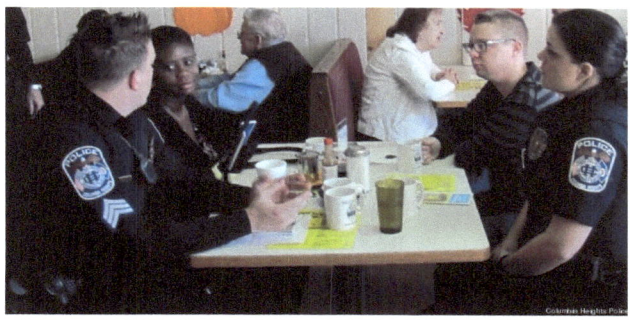

COLUMBIA HEIGHTS POLICE DEPARTMENT SGTS. JUSTIN PLETCHER AND MAGGIE TITUS SPEAK WITH RESIDENTS DURING A RECENT COFFEE WITH A COP SESSION. (PHOTO: COLUMBIA HEIGHTS POLICE DEPARTMENT)

Through the programs Nadeau has implemented, police hope to gain the trust of residents. But the officers themselves may also come away with a better view of community members.

"Law enforcement officers, many times, end up having ... a jaded view of police and community contacts just because of all the negative experiences that they have as a result of just doing their jobs," Nadeau said. "I think that having these positive interactions ... helps them to maybe refocus somewhat on the fact that the majority of the people in our community are great citizens and

those relationships are important to both sides."

Building trust between police and the community has to start from an early age.

When Nadeau first came to Columbia Heights, youth crime rates were high, and a school board member told him that police had an especially rocky relationship with kids. Now, under Nadeau's leadership, a major focus of the city's community policing efforts is on youth. The department offers a variety of programs -- from open gym hours to one-on-one mentoring – and officers visit each first-, second-, third- and fourth-grade classroom in the city's schools at least once a school year, building community trust from an early age. Since 2008, juvenile arrests in Columbia Heights have dropped by more than half. (Nationwide, juvenile arrest rates also fell during this period, though not as steeply.)

Officer visits to classrooms give students a chance to see "that familiar face, that this is a person that works in our community that cares about kids and families," said Michele DeWitt, principal of Highland Elementary

School. This, she noted, is particularly important for students who have had negative experiences with law enforcement, like seeing family members be arrested.

Nadeau approached DeWitt a few years ago about the possibility of police doing more youth outreach. They started by getting the department involved in a bullying prevention program, in which officers would read anti-bullying books and discuss them with classes. The mentoring program followed soon after. And there's the annual visit when police let kids check out squad cars -- not surprisingly, a student favorite.

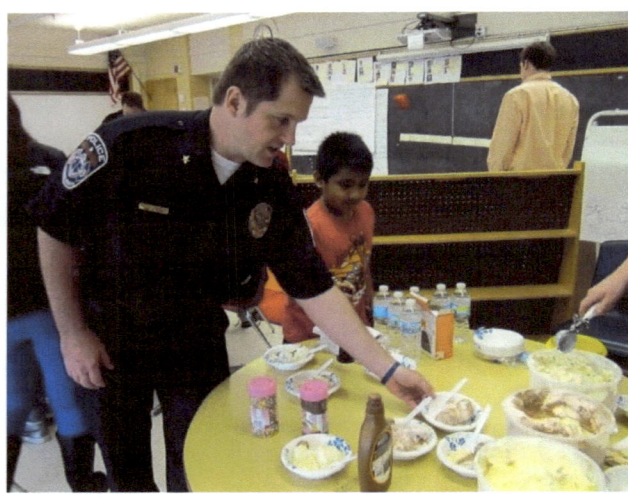

POLICE CHIEF SCOTT NADEAU CELEBRATES THE END OF THE 2012-2013 SCHOOL YEAR WITH THE STUDENT HE

MENTORS AT HIGHLAND. (PHOTO: COLUMBIA HEIGHTS POLICE DEPARTMENT)

"It was a really concerted effort," DeWitt said of Nadeau's school involvement initiatives. "It wasn't just, 'Let's try this and then we'll move on and try something else,' it was the police chief really thinking outside the box and saying, 'What can we do to just inundate this community with a positive message?'"

Nadeau himself mentors a student once a week. He said that when police would walk into schools several years ago, they were greeted with alarm from teachers and fear from students, who saw their presence as a sign that something was wrong.

"Now when we walk down the hallways, the teachers smile, they're happy that you're there," the police chief said. "I probably get about 50 to 60 high-fives from some of the kids in the school. The fact that it's no longer unusual to see police officers in the schools has fundamentally changed our relationships with these kids."

Many local departments adopted community policing in response to a federal push in the 1990s.

By the 1990s, the philosophy of community policing had become widely known in law enforcement. DOJ's Community Oriented Policing Services office was formed in 1994 as part of President Bill Clinton's sweeping crime package. Created to support local agencies' community policing efforts, COPS sought to get 100,000 officers hired and distribute billions in grants. COPS Principal Deputy Director Sandra Webb told HuffPost that the office has provided community policing funding for about 70 percent of law enforcement agencies nationwide.

But while community policing can and does occur without federal support, Webb explained that attention for COPS' efforts waned after Clinton's initial investment, and the department's budget declined significantly, from a high of $1.6 billion in 1998 to just $208 million for 2015. (In 2009, $550 million was budgeted, but the stimulus package also allocated a separate one-time $1 billion for hiring officers). The George W. Bush administration actually proposed completely eliminating the COPS program in all eight of its annual budget proposals,

though it was never successful in accomplishing that.

Number of community policing officers peaks sharply in 2000

In the late 1990s, the number of local police departments using dedicated community policing officers increased dramatically -- from 34 percent in 1997 to 66 percent in 2000 -- but that same percentage plummeted in the years after.

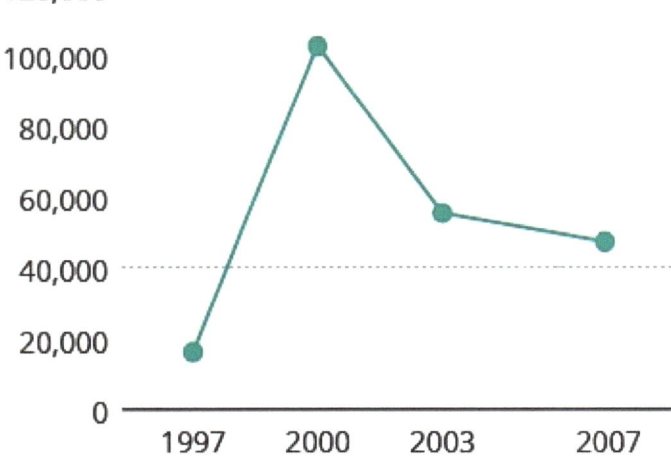

Number of officers (rounded to the nearest 1,000)

Source: U.S. Department of Justice, Bureau of Justice Statistics

According to a Justice Department survey, the late 1990s saw a marked increase in the number of dedicated community policing officers specifically tasked with building relationships in their assigned neighborhoods: In 1997, 34 percent of all departments used such officers, while by 2000, the number had jumped to 66 percent. Similarly, there were 17,000 dedicated community policing officers in local departments in 1997, compared to 103,000 in 2000. But the survey found that starting in 2000, the number of community policing officers began to decline sharply, and had dropped by more than half by 2007.

But aggressive policing tactics gradually became more commonplace.

Mike Scott, director and founder of the Center for Problem-Oriented Policing, says that by the turn of the millennium, a confluence of factors had contributed to a turn away from a community-oriented approach toward more aggressive policing.

These included the gradual militarization of even small local departments, which began to use SWAT team-style tactics more regularly, as well as a tougher response to political protests in light of the violent showdown between police and protesters at the 1999 World Trade Organization meeting in

Seattle. Police also began to rely more on strategies associated with the war on drugs, such as stop-and-frisk. In addition, "broken windows" policing, a controversial approach in which police departments aggressively pursue low-level crime, became more common in the late 1990s. Finally, after the Sept. 11 terrorist attacks, federal funds previously devoted to community policing programs were redirected to fund counterterrorism and surveillance efforts.

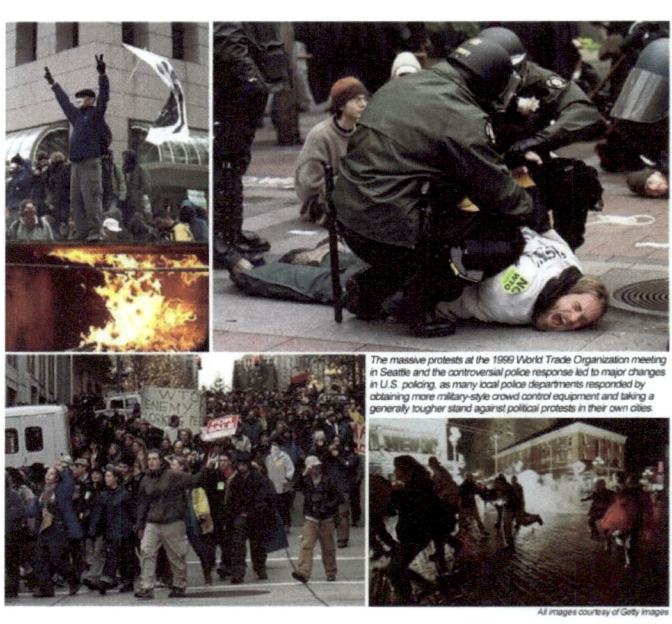

The massive protests at the 1999 World Trade Organization meeting in Seattle and the controversial police response led to major changes in U.S. policing, as many local police departments responded by obtaining more military-style crowd control equipment and taking a generally tougher stand against political protests in their own cities

All images courtesy of Getty Images

Starting in 2008, the Great Recession also contributed to the shift, with many police departments seeing slashed budgets -- in Redlands, for example, department staff was cut by a third. Once the federal support for community policing began to disappear, Scott argues, many cash-strapped departments that were less invested in the concept turned their attention to areas where more federal dollars were coming in, particularly counterterrorism and disaster preparedness. Cities like Redlands, which were genuinely interested in community policing, didn't change their philosophies, though they had to carry them out with fewer resources.

Though many law enforcement agencies have turned to more aggressive strategies, they haven't necessarily created safer communities or better relationships.

The result, Scott says, was a rise in aggressive policing that eroded much of the progress that community policing had made, particularly among minorities. As critics of "broken windows" have pointed out, there is little evidence that aggressive policing has made most communities significantly safer.

Scott argues that the coexistence of community policing and the aggressive approach grew increasingly "schizophrenic," essentially canceling each other out. A department's community policing arm might take a softer, problem-solving approach in a neighborhood during the day, only to have that goodwill undone by SWAT-style tactics in the same neighborhood that same night.

"If we've learned nothing else over 200 years or so of policing, it's that police will never gain either the trust of the public or improve their personal safety solely by aggressive policing," Scott said. "It's a failed strategy. It's a natural kind of reaction, but it's the wrong reaction."

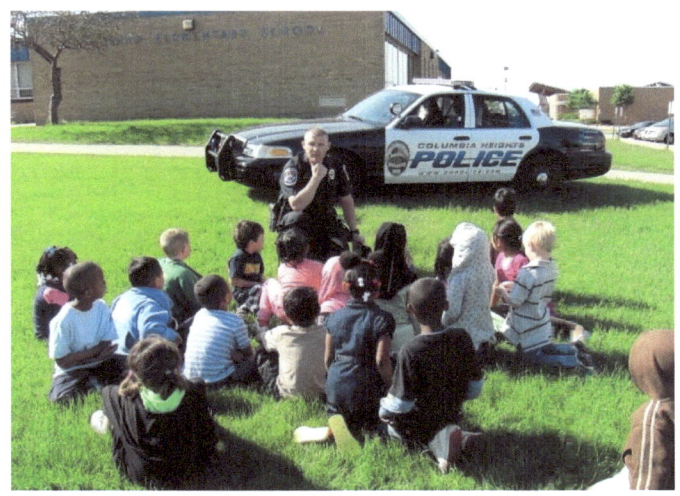

SCOTT NADEAU HOPES MEETING WITH STUDENTS YEAR AFTER YEAR -- HERE, AN OFFICER READS WITH A GROUP OF ELEMENTARY SCHOOL STUDENTS -- WILL HELP BUILD COMMUNITY TRUST. (PHOTO: COLUMBIA HEIGHTS POLICE DEPARTMENT)

With a renewed focus on community policing, plenty of cities can serve as models for others looking to adopt the philosophy.

The Justice Department has acknowledged the problem: Amid protests over Brown's and Garner's deaths, DOJ last fall announced the launch of a newthree-year initiative to study racial bias in the criminal justice system and restore community trust in the police. In December, President Barack Obama again called for investment in community policing, proposing a $260 million funding package that would in part go toward providing training and resources for police reform.

Across the country, many local police departments are also renewing their efforts to change the way they interact with communities. When the U.S. Conference of Mayors convened last month, it addressed the deaths of Brown and Garner and issued recommendations that cities use community policing to improve residents' trust. From Chatham, New Jersey, to Sacramento, California, police departments are testing out new ways to improve their relationships with the communities they serve. Redlands is one of the places where the community approach has become a fundamental part of policing. In 1993, then-Police Captain Jim Bueermann was tasked with overseeing a transition from traditional to community-oriented policing in response to strained relations between the department and the public.

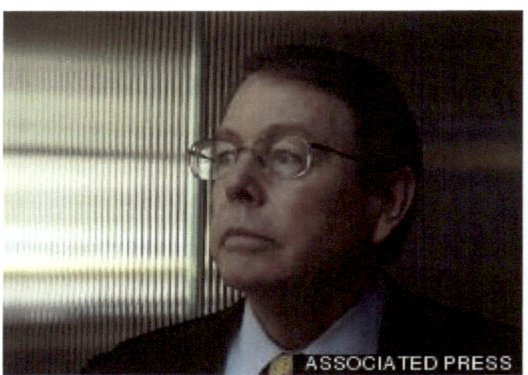

JIM BUEERMANN. (PHOTO: ALEX BRANDON/AP)

Bueermann, who became police chief in 1998 and served until 2011, was known for the partnerships he made and his heavy reliance on evidence-driven strategies. Under his leadership, Redlands' housing, recreation and senior services departments were consolidated into the police department as part of a program to identify risks for young people. Though the city eventually separated the departments again, the collaboration -- involving schools, hospitals, the probation department and businesses -- gave police the ability to make quality-of-life services and crime prevention a core part of their community policing approach.

"Police and community have to co-produce public safety," said Bueerman, who now heads a nonprofit dedicated to innovations in policing. "That's probably one of the strongest pieces of community policing that frequently gets missed by practitioners. They have to reach out to the community and say ... 'How are we, all of us, going to solve this problem?'"

Ed Gomez, a history professor who has lived in Redlands for 11 years, commends Bueermann for promoting peace, balance and trust in the community. Gomez chairs the city's Human Relations Commission, a volunteer advisory board that works with city officials to address residents' concerns and protect their rights. The board, Gomez said, doesn't often hear complaints about the police department. Gomez believes current Chief Mark Garcia, who took over from Bueermann in 2011, has continued his predecessor's legacy. But, he cautioned, community trust can't be taken for granted.

"That's something that will go away if it's not held sacred by the citizens and the police department itself," Gomez said. "I believe Chief Garcia is doing what he can to keep things in place the way they were, so I hope he will continue that and maybe even take a more active role. It will also be up to the community to hold his feet to the fire."

Current officers say they're dedicated to continuing a legacy of trust with residents.

"I think the community has a high expectation of us, and we have a high expectation of them back," Redlands Police Commander Chris Catren said. "When significant crime, especially, occurs, their expectation is that we're going to do everything we can to solve it, and our expectation

41

conversely is that they're going to assist us, and they do."

And when tragedy does strike, it's easier for the community to recover when everyone is working together.

Redlands' approach was put to the test when Gail Howard's son and three others boys were shot in an unprovoked attack at a playground. Throughout the subsequent investigation, police treated the shooting as a tragedy not just for the victims and their families, but also for the department.

"Lt. Mike Reiss told me that night at the hospital, 'This is personal, they shotMY son, they shot MY boy'" Howard said. Reiss had been a football coach for Jordan before the shooting. Jordan, now 20, is healthy and still plays football.

The week after the shooting, the police department partnered with faith groups to lead a vigil for the victims. About a thousand people marched alongside officers from the location of the shooting to nearby Micah House, an after-school program for at-risk kids and one of the police department's partner organizations.

"The fact that they pulled together and put on a march right afterwards showed a desire to pull the community together, and it did pull the community together," said Dianna Lawson, a Micah House program coordinator. "It just made a difference."

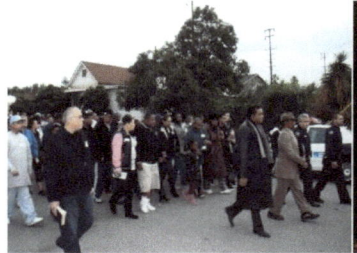 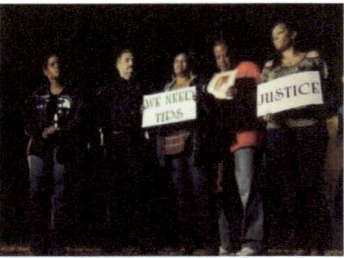

LEFT: HUNDREDS GATHERED TO MARCH FOR PEACE AFTER THE 2011 REDLANDS SHOOTING. (PHOTO: MICAH HOUSE). RIGHT: FOR THE ONE-YEAR ANNIVERSARY OF THE SHOOTING, AT WHICH POINT THE KILLERS HAD NOT YET BEEN FOUND, CHIEF MARK GARCIA JOINED THE VICTIMS' MOTHERS IN ASKING THE PUBLIC TO COME FORWARD WITH ANY INFORMATION. (PHOTO: GAIL HOWARD)

Community policing means working proactively and building relationships in the face of tension and issues.

In the aftermath of the shooting, there was concern from residents that police weren't dedicating enough resources to the area where the incident occurred, on Redlands' north side, which Gomez described as the historically poor part of the city. Garcia said the department responded by increasing their presence in the neighborhood, stationing a community policing officer at Micah House and conducting regular meetings with local citizen groups to exchange information.

And though Howard was appreciative of the police's efforts, as the investigation dragged on, some of the relatives of the other victims accused the department of not putting enough work into the case. Howard said they and some others in the black community believed the case was not getting sufficient attention because the victims were black. She thinks this notion is false, though she acknowledged that Redlands' efforts hadn't fully erased minorities' distrust of police.

' I do feel like I'm in the middle of something, that a lot of people in the black community want me to actually hate the police, and not like the police, but I cannot feel that way," she said, referencing the national protests over police brutality. "You've got to understand where I've been and how much they've done for me."

Since her son's close call, Howard's relationship with police has helped her find ways to get more involved in the community. She took charge of theShop with a Cop program, which allows needy kids to go holiday shopping while fostering relationships between children and police officers. "Some of these kids, the only contact they have with police is seeing their parent be wrestled down to the ground and handcuffed, and we want them to know that there's good officers out there. ... I want kids not to be afraid to approach that police officer," Howard said.

Each year since the shooting, Howard has held a vigil to remember the victims. She noted that the police chief or members of the force have attended every march.

But building trust isn't easy for minority groups who have long felt the police have failed them.

Even amid the best of intentions, the shift away from traditional policing can be difficult to implement. Perhaps the biggest obstacle to the community policing approach is fostering trust among minority groups.

A 2014 Pew Research poll found that while most Americans hold a generally favorable view of their local police, blacks and Latinos have much less faith in their police forces than white Americans do.

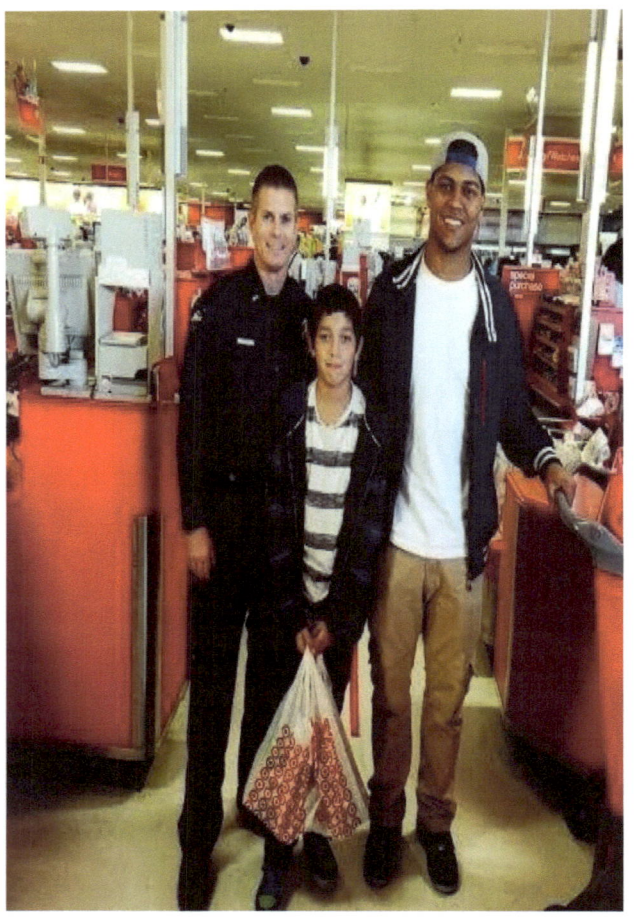

LT. MIKE REISS, JORDAN HOWARD AND A SHOP WITH A COP STUDENT. (PHOTO: GAIL HOWARD)

"The crazy thing about it is at the end, you see the officers giving the kids their phone numbers, 'If you need something or someone to talk to, give me a call,'" she added. "And to me, that's a success, because now it's personal."

Good Cop, Bad Cop

How much confidence do you have in police officers in your community...

...to do a good job of enforcing the law?

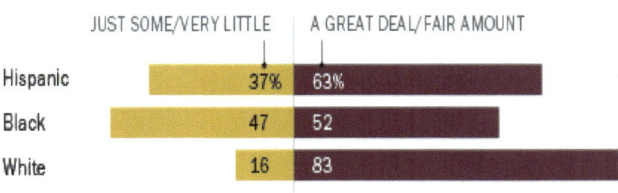

	JUST SOME/VERY LITTLE	A GREAT DEAL/FAIR AMOUNT
Hispanic	37%	63%
Black	47	52
White	16	83

...to not use excessive force on suspects?

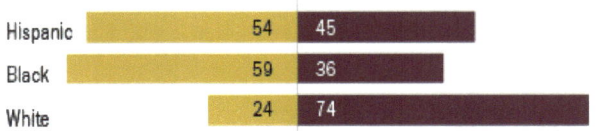

Hispanic	54	45
Black	59	36
White	24	74

...to treat Hispanics and whites equally?

Hispanic	51	46
Black	55	41
White	25	72

...to treat blacks and whites equally?

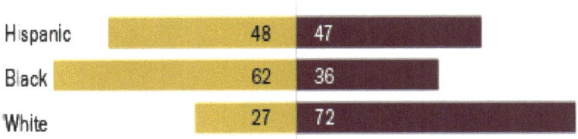

Hispanic	48	47
Black	62	36
White	27	72

Note: Survey conducted Aug. 20-24, 2014. Voluntary responses of "None" and "Don't know/Refused" not shown. Blacks and whites include only non-Hispanics. Hispanics are of any race.

Source: Pew Research Center/USA Today

PEW RESEARCH CENTER

Pew Research Center

Bridging that gap by reaching out to minority groups is a key part of community policing, and the Columbia Heights police department has made it a priority. Dana Caraway, a pastoral assistant at the multicultural Church of Nations, said that her church has a robust relationship with local police. But it's difficult to surmount the historic tensions that some minority groups perceive between racial justice and the very institution of policing. The pervasiveness of those tensions came to the surface in Columbia Heights several years ago, when the Church of Nations discovered that minority members felt uncomfortable about the presence of patrol officers idling in the church parking lot.

The city of Madison, Wisconsin, began implementing community policing in the early 1980s. At that time, David Couper, who served as Madison's chief of police from 1972 until 1993, pushed his department to work in a more community-oriented, decentralized way, and also sought to diversify what was then a mostly white, entirely male department. Couper essentially invented what has been dubbed in some circles as the **"Madison way"** of community policing. Under his watch, the first officer focused on community policing took to the streets of Madison.

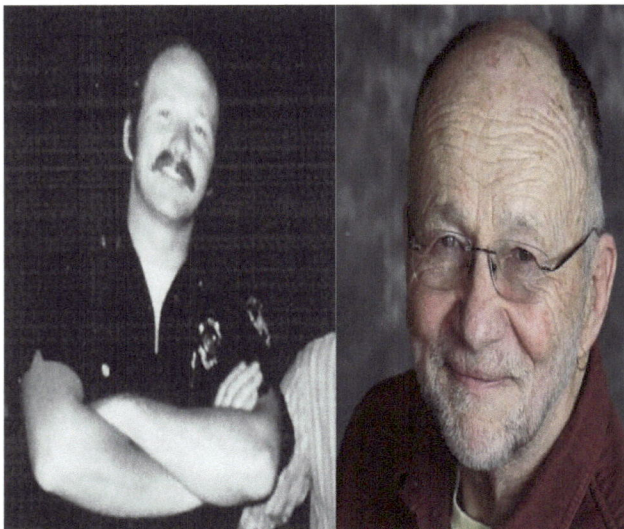

DAVID COUPER

Today, the department maintains a number of community policing initiatives, including a citizen police academy, black and Latino youth academies, teams of mental health officers and community policing teams dedicated to each of the city's neighborhoods. An "Amigos en Azul" team works in the department's Hispanic-majority South District to erode the barriers between officers and the city's Latino residents.

But although the department was an early adopter of community policing and has been heralded as a success story, statistics show the Wisconsin

capital still has a long way to go. The city has an overwhelmingly high disparity between arrest rates of black and white residents, with black residents estimated to be nine times more likely to be arrested than whites.

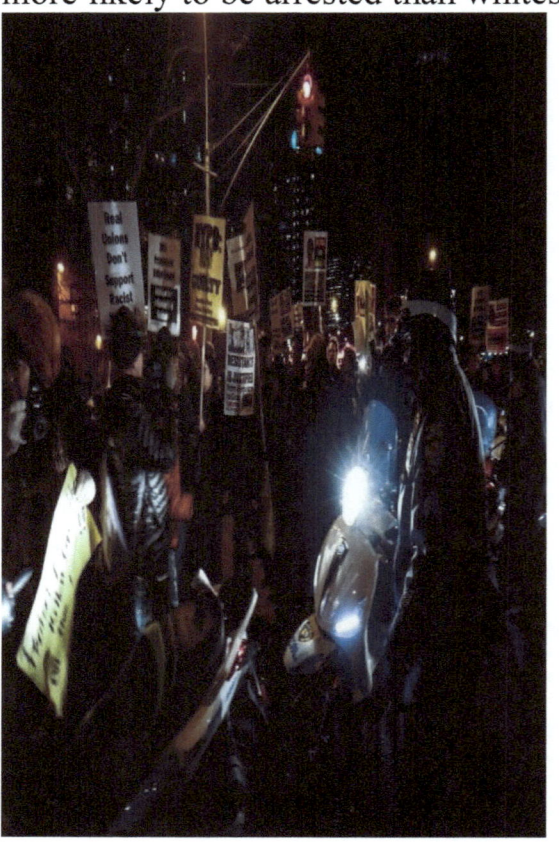

NEW YORKERS PROTEST IN DECEMBER 2014 AFTER GRAND JURIES INVESTIGATING THE DEATHS OF MICHAEL BROWN AND ERIC GARNER FAILED TO INDICT THE POLICE OFFICERS INVOLVED. (PHOTO: CEM

OZDEL/ANADOLU
AGENCY/GETTY IMAGES)

Some solutions may be perceived negatively by those for whom police mistrust is difficult to discard.

reflect the values of community control and self-determination."

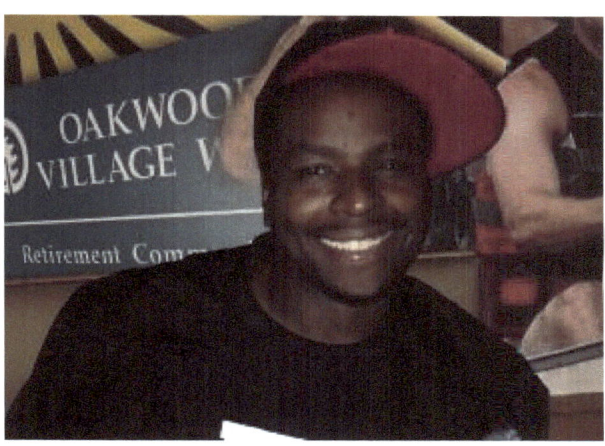

ANTHONY WARD

That disparity was at the heart of an open letter penned last month by an activist group called the Young, Black and Gifted Coalition, which discussed the issue of arrest rates as well as the deaths of Brown and Garner.

In the letter, the group criticized Madison's community policing efforts as ineffective, called for vast reforms to the local criminal justice system and outlined its preferred form of policing in minority neighborhoods: None whatsoever. "Although Madison's model of community policing and attempt to build trust between the community and police, even acting as 'social workers,' may be a step above certain other communities, our arrest rates and incarceration disparities still top the nation," the letter read. "Our ultimate goal is finding alternatives to incarceration and policing, and our steps forward as a community should

Anthony Ward, a former Madison police officer who now works with at-risk African-American boys, acknowledged that the department has its heart in the right place when it comes to using community policing in minority neighborhoods. But in practice, he argued, the strategy results in a much higher number of officers in squad cars driving through communities of color and poor areas, which Ward believes sends a strong message to residents.

"While community policing sounds fine and dandy, what is actually happening is community seizing," Ward said. "We're not saying we won't call the police when we need help, but people in minority neighborhoods don't need to see them every time we look over our shoulder as if the community doesn't know how to take care of themselves, like we're savages and need a police presence to be civilized."

Mike Koval, Madison's current chief of police, admitted that his department has played an undeniable role in minority communities' negative impressions of the way people of color are policed. However, Koval said that instead of pulling back at this tense moment, he wants his department to "double down" on its commitment to a community-oriented approach. He thinks the time is right for officers to take on the role of problem solvers, rather than simply law enforcers.

"Right now, it's almost a calculus of a perfect storm for when community policing can really make some inroads on rebuilding some community trust," Koval said. "To me, this only creates an even greater challenge for our officers to prove our critics wrong."

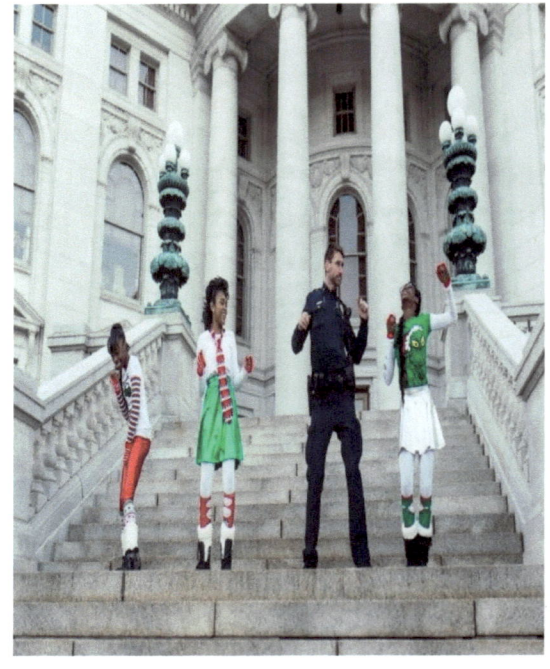

A MADISON POLICE OFFICER JOINS A GROUP OF GIRLS FROM THE LOCAL BOYS & GIRLS CLUB FILMING A VIDEO ON THE STEPS OF THE WISCONSIN STATE CAPITOL IN DECEMBER 2014. COMMUNITY POLICING ADVOCATES SAY THAT POSITIVE INTERACTIONS WITH THE COMMUNITY, EVEN ONES AS SIMPLE AS THIS, CAN GO A LONG WAY. (PHOTO: MADISON POLICE DEPARTMENT)

Ward hopes the department will do a better job pairing officers with neighborhoods they genuinely care about and ensuring that all officers are trained in cultural awareness. Only then, he said, can an effective partnership between communities of color and police officers be formed and the disparity in arrest rates and community trust be meaningfully addressed.

"I believe minority groups are going to be the ones who are going to change our community, who are going to make it better and we can do that in conjunction with police officers, but not with them at the helm," he said.

It's a difficult task, but the conditions are ripe for change.

Like some of the skeptics in Madison, Tometi, the #BlackLivesMatter co-founder, is hesitant to embrace community policing, which she describes as "a euphemism for more surveillance" of minority communities. Tometi considers community policing on its own to be "empty rhetoric," unless it is accompanied by meaningful

community investment and the altogether rejection of "broken windows" policing. She is hopeful that the demonstrations led by #BlackLivesMatter and other groups can help inspire such reform.

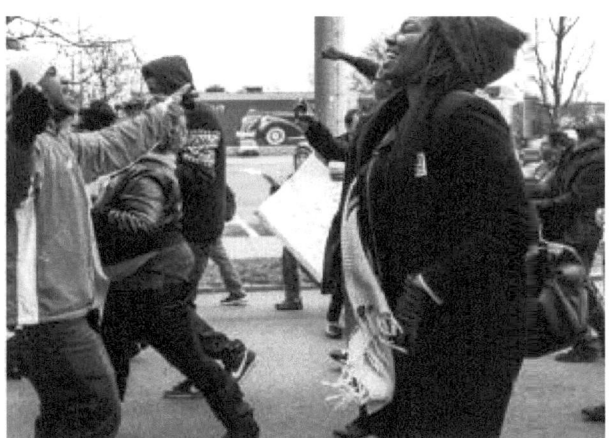

OPAL TOMETI

"Training will not help if officers do not have a fundamental shift in how they understand their roles as public servants, not as racial profiling agents," Tometi said. "For us, an end to broken windows is healing. Community investment is healing. Not more police or policing technologies for more surveillance and racial profiling."

Despite the challenges, some experts are cautiously optimistic for change.

Couper, who today is an Episcopal priest and maintains the blog **"Improving Police,"** said he is hopeful some departments with "wise leaders and probably wise mayors in their cities" will take advantage of what he sees as an opportunity for police to take a new approach. "We're at a position where we can take the more comfortable way and the way we do that is to maintain the status quo. The argument for the status quo is they haven't done anything wrong and to wait until it blows over," Couper said. "Or, we can show some leadership and ask: Why is it that we're so mistrusted, why are we losing support and blaming the messenger on this?"

"Change is (hopefully) coming, but from my experience it will take a long, long time," Couper said later, when asked specifically about the racial tensions in Madison. "But why not start now?"

MADISON'S COMMUNITY POLICING OFFICERS ENGAGE WITH RESIDENTS IN A NUMBER OF COMMUNITY EVENTS THROUGHOUT THE YEAR -- BUT CRITICS SAY SUCH EFFORTS FALL FAR SHORT OF THE SORT OF REFORM NEEDED IN THE WISCONSIN CAPITAL. (PHOTO: MADISON POLICE DEPARTMENT)

And sometimes even small gestures end up going a long way.

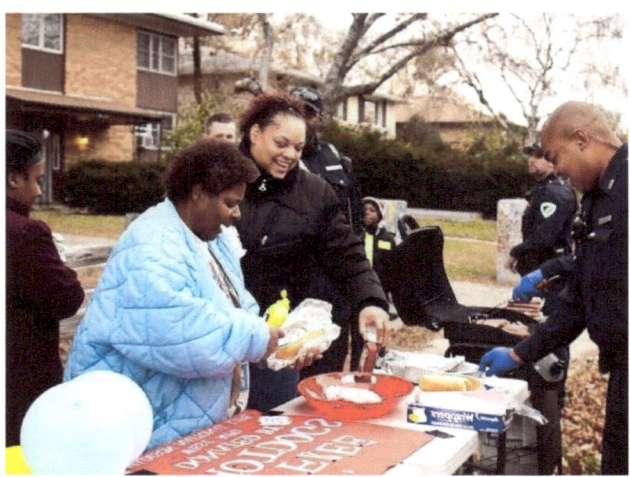

"You can't always solve them, but people need to see police trying to solve the problems that the people who live there regard as problems, to see them working on their behalf as opposed to pursuing their own interests or something else," said Cordner, the Kutztown professor. "You can't just repaint the police cars or hire a new police chief."

"Policing is frequently not pleasant, sometimes it's very complicated and just messy," Bueermann said. "A police department's ability to weather a controversial incident -- it's almost always involving use of force -- is a direct function of the trust and confidence the public has in that department."

Nadeau acknowledged that the national focus on police brutality and mistreatment of minorities has had an effect on residents' impressions of police in Columbia Heights. But he believes that a fundamental part of his job is to engage those concerns, and to actually implement the feedback he gets. So, when Caraway told police that residents were responding negatively to officers idling in the church parking lot, the department ended the practice and met with the congregation to address the concerns. It was a small act, but an example of the philosophy that, over time, may be one of the best chances to repair the damaged relationships between police and the public.

ARE POLICE IN YOUR COMMUNITY MAKING UNIQUE EFFORTS TO INSPIRE CHANGE AND IMPROVE RELATIONSHIPS? WE WANT TO HEAR ABOUT IT.

WHAT COLOR IS YOUR PERSONALITY?

BY BENJAMIN BIRELY

COLOR PSYCHOLOGY TELLS US THAT OUR INSTINCTIVE COLOR PREFERENCES REVEAL THE DEEPEST PARTS OF OUR PERSONALITIES. WHAT COLOR DO YOU SUBCONSCIOUSLY RELATE TO?

This is my personality color after I took the quiz or I entered to play the color personality choices.
EddieAdel
Managing Editor,
My Connections magazine

You can use the link below the image to connect to the personality game colors, or you can go to myconnectionsmagazine.com and look for the article; "What color is your personality, Let's play".

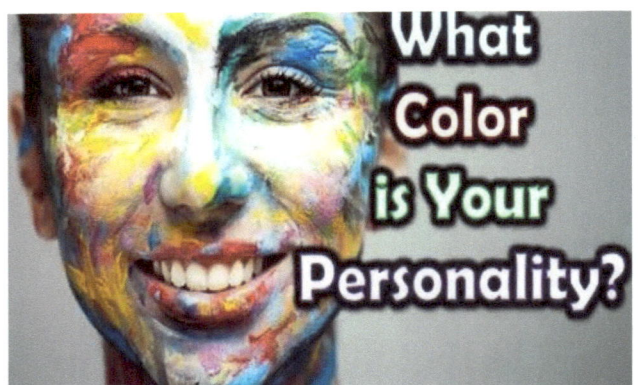

What Color is Your Personality?

Color psychology tells us that our instinctive color preferences reveal the deepest parts of our personalities. What color do you subconsciously relate to?

WWW.ARTICLESBASE.COM

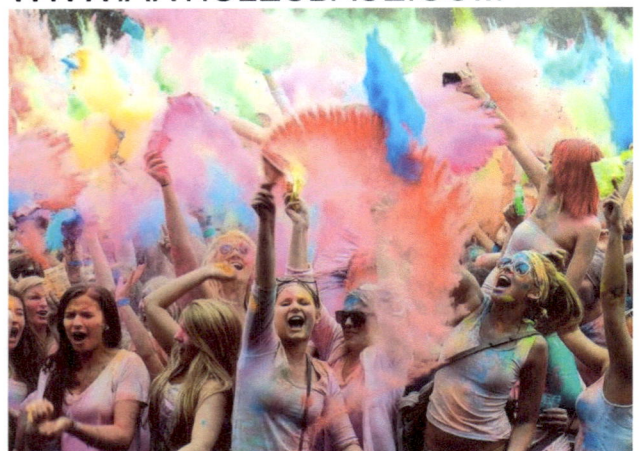

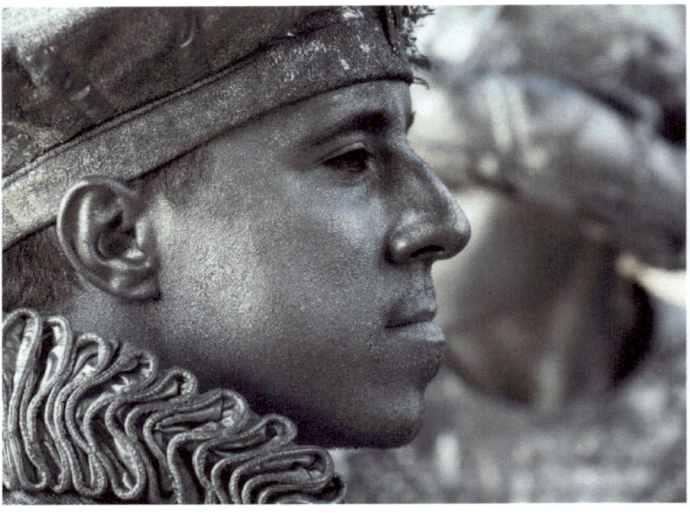

You belong to the silver family! The color psychology quiz tells us that you subconsciously most relate to those silvers, whites, and greys. First off, feel very unique! This is a rare color family to belong to, and it means that you're super special and, obviously, super interesting. This group of colors is frequently associated with purity and spirituality. You exist on a higher plane than most of us and you're deeply connected to spirituality. This can manifest itself in many ways. Maybe you're religious, maybe you love philosophy, maybe Zen meditation is your thing, or perhaps you simply enjoy a clean, simple and drama free life. Regardless of which category fits you, you're above a lot of the messy things in life and you seek balance and peace. You're a rare breed.

What do you think about being such a highly evolved silver soul? Tell us in the comments!

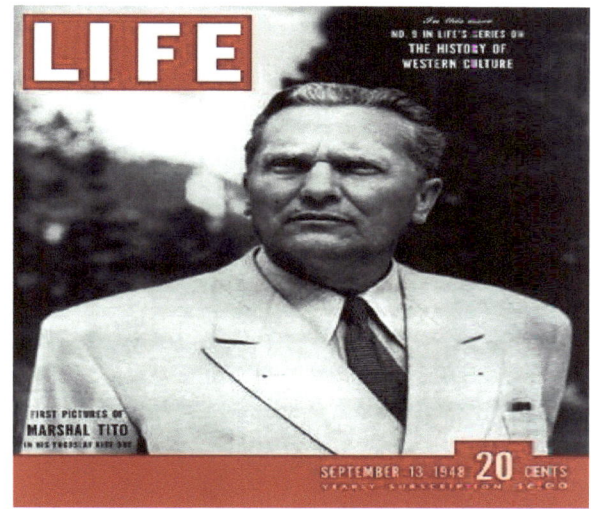

RELATED MAGAZINES

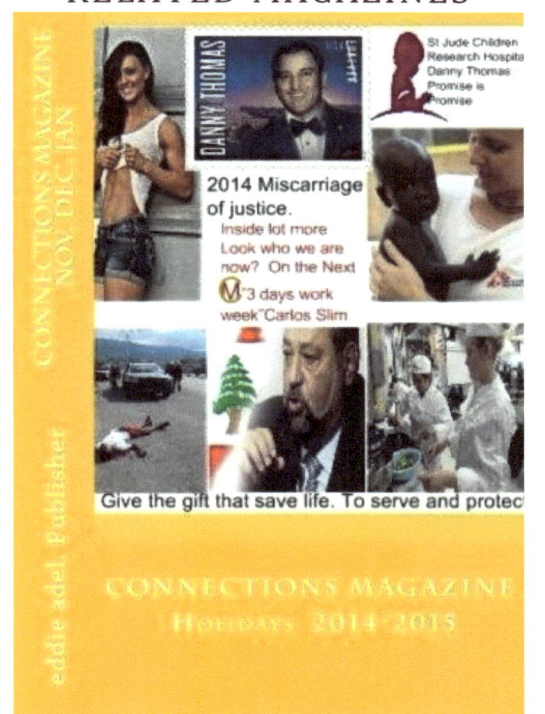

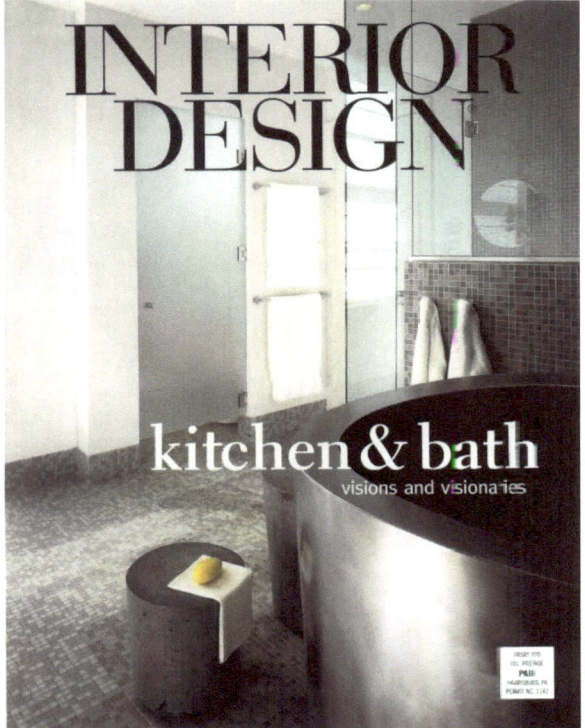

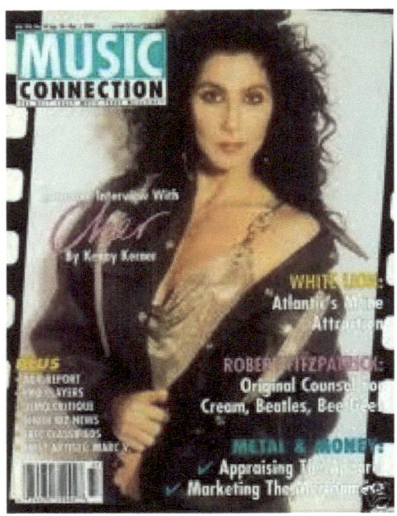

HEALTH AND SAFETY USING VARIETY HOT TUBS JACUZZI AT HOME AND ANYWHERE ELSE

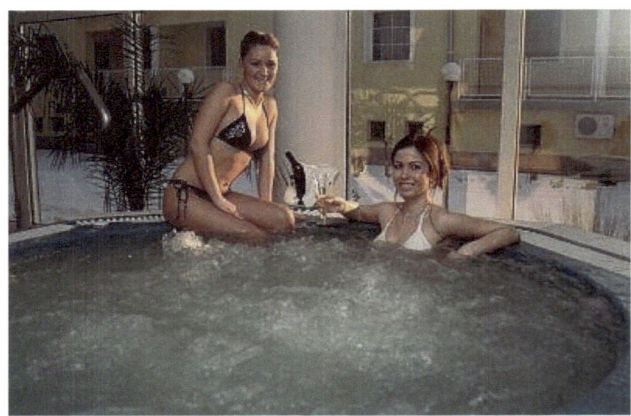

Maintain Sanitizer & Water Balance

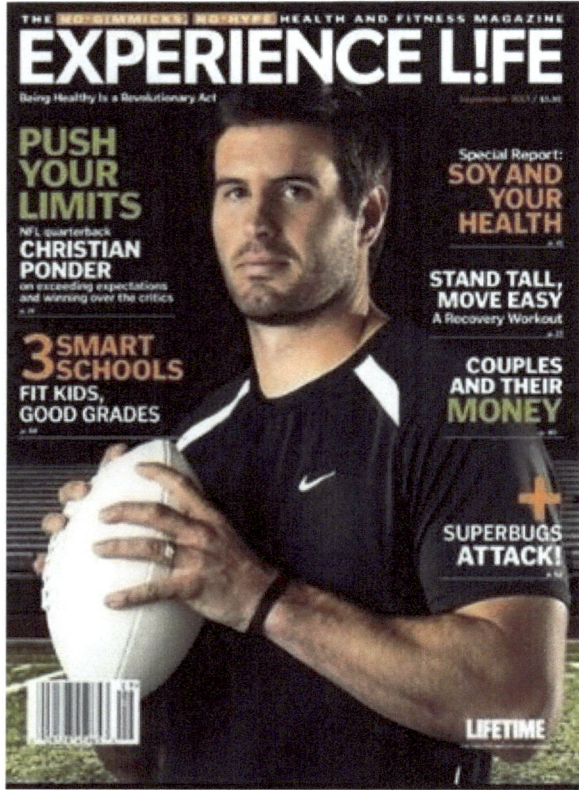

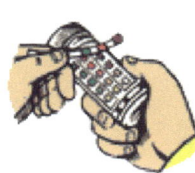 Do not enter a hot tub unless you know that the sanitizer level is adequate to keep the water healthy and free of harmful microorganisms. Maintaining the Total Alkalinity (TA) and pH for proper water balance, and regular shocking of the water will make your sanitizer much more effective in controlling

bacteria.

Use the appropriate test strips to monitor TA and pH, as well as the sanitizer level. A newbacteria test is also now available.

Chemicals & Spa Supplies

Chemicals, additives and cleaning compounds are best kept in a cool, dry, and well ventilated location, away from direct sunlight and out of the reach of children. Read and follow all directions on chemical labels.

As a rule, spa chemicals should not be mixed together prior to addition to the water. Dissolve dry chemicals one at a time in a plastic bucket of clean water, then pour into the hot tub. This will also prevent damage to the acrylic shell (or PVC liner) from direct contact of un-dissolved granules.

Alcohol and Drugs

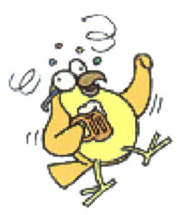
Hot water amplifies the effects of alcohol and certain drugs, and the result can be dangerous. Consult your doctor regarding the use of prescription drugs. Many people prefer the enjoyment of a chilled soft drink, juice or mineral water while relaxing in their spas.

Water Temperature

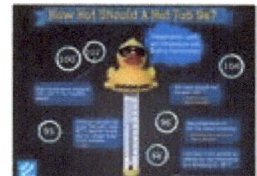
Soaking for too long in elevated water temperatures can raise body heat to hazardous levels. The National Spa and Pool Institute considers 104° F to be the maximum safe water temperature for adults, and modern spas are normally set at the factory not to exceed that limit.

A safe soaking time should not exceed 15 minutes. Some medical authorities have recommended a lower maximum temperature of 100° to 102° F. They advise that since infants and children are more sensitive to heat, they should be exposed to water of not more than 95° F, for no more than 10 minutes. Consult with your family doctor.

Persons with heart disease, diabetes, high or low blood pressure, or any other serious illness should not enter a spa or hot tub without first consulting with, and obtaining the advice of a physician.

Keeping a floating thermometer in the water is a good idea, especially if your spa does not have a digital temperature readout indicator.

Children and Infants

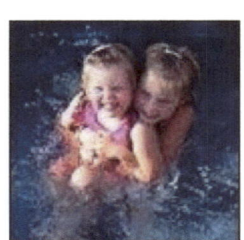

Children should be introduced into the hot tub or spa slowly to give them time to adjust to the change in temperature and to alleviate fear or discomfort. Infants should not enter a hot tub without

doctor's approval.

NEVER, UNDER ANY CIRCUMSTANCES leave children unattended in hot tubs, spas or pools. Even shallow ones pose a drowning hazard, and even a few moments alone is too long. *Better safe than sorry* is a good rule to tub by!

Pregnancy

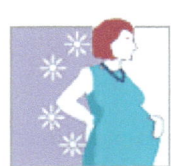

Pregnant women should not enter a hot tub or spa without first consulting with their physician and following the doctor's advice.

Hair Entanglement

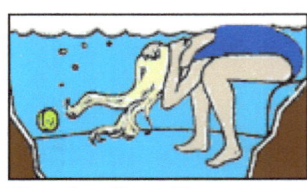

Drain Suction

A drowning risk can occur when a bather's hair becomes entangled in a drain cover, as the water and hair are drawn through the drain. Never allow children (or anyone) to play with heads underwater in a spa.

The U.S. Consumer Product Safety Commission helped develop a standard requiring dome-shaped drain outlets and two outlets for each pump. This reduces the powerful suction if one drain is blocked. Consumers with older spas should have new drain covers installed and may want to consider getting a spa with two drains to help prevent entrapment. If you have a swimming pool, have it checked as well.

Regularly have a professional check your spa or hot tub and make sure it is in good, safe working condition, and that drain covers are in place and not cracked or missing. Check the drain covers yourself throughout the year. Make sure you have a GFCI-protected power disconnect device installed, and know where and how to use it in an emergency.

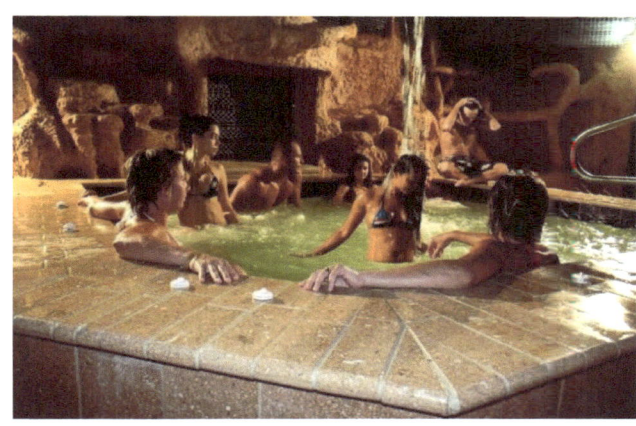

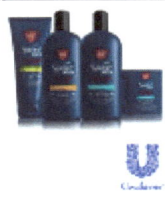

OFFER OF THE *WEEK*

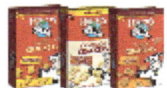

BUY 1 GET 1 FREE (UP TO $4.29)

HORIZON®

Any Horizon® Snack Crackers, Sandwich Crackers or Snack Grahams

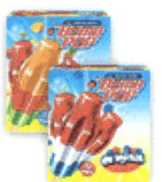

SAVE 75¢

BOMB POP®

on any one (1) carton Bomb Pop® Frozen Novelty

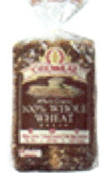

SAVE $1.00

OROWEAT

on any one (1) Oroweat bread variety

JOIN·OUR MAILING LIST

& never miss a great coupon.
Sign Up

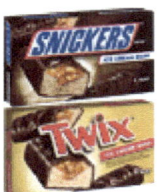

SAVE $1.00

MARS ICE CREAM

on any ONE (1) SNICKERS®, TWIX®, M&M'S®, MILKY WAY® or DOVEBAR® Brand Ice Cream Multi-Packs (3ct.-6ct.)

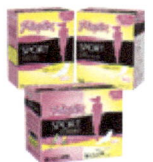

SAVE $3.00

PLAYTEX® SPORT®

on any One (1) Playtex® Sport® Pads, Liners or Combo Pack (excludes 16ct, 18ct Pad and 20ct liner)

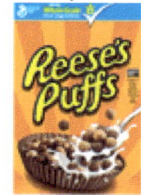

SAVE 50¢ ON ONE

BIG G CEREALS®

when you buy ONE BOX Reese's Puffs cereal

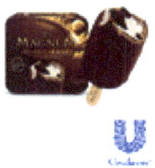

SAVE $0.75

MAGNUM®

on any ONE (1) Magnum® Ice Cream Bar Multipack

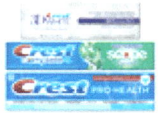

$1.50 OFF

CREST®

TWO Crest® Toothpastes 3.0 oz or more or Liquid Gel (excludes Crest® Cavity, Baking Soda, Tartar Control, and trial/travel size)

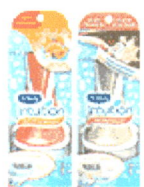

SAVE $3.00

SCHICK® INTUITION®

on any one (1) Schick® Intuition® Razor

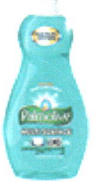

SAVE $0.25

PALMOLIVE®

On any Palmolive® Liquid Dish Soap

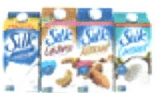

SAVE $0.75

SILK®

off any One (1) Silk® Half Gallon

EXPLORE THIS WEEK'S SAVINGS

TARGET WEEKLY AD

Find all the best deals at your Target store.

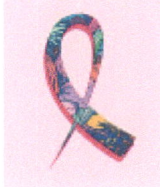

YOU SHOP, WE GIVE

BCRF

We'll donate 10% of what you spend to fund breast cancer research.

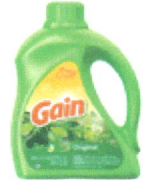

$1.00 OFF
GAIN®

ONE Gain® Laundry Detergent 40 oz or larger liquid or 22 load or larger powder (excludes Fireworks and trial/travel size)

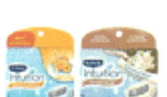

SAVE $4.00
SCHICK® INTUITION®

on any one (1) Schick® Intuition® Refill

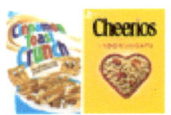

SAVE $1.00 ON TWO
BIG G CEREALS®

when you buy TWO BOXES any flavor General Mills Big G cereals: Cheerios™ • Cinnamon Toast Crunch™ • Chex™...

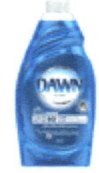

25¢ OFF
DAWN®

ONE Dawn® product (excludes trial/travel size)

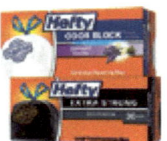

SAVE $1.00
HEFTY® TRASH BAGS

off any ONE (1) package of Hefty® Trash Bags

FREE CLASSIFIEDS ONLINE AT ANAHEIMPUBLISHING.CO

1. **AA-AMERICA ANYWHERE-BUY/SELL AND OTHER SERVICES.**
   anaheimpublishing.co/

   Free Classifieds Published By *ANAHEIMPUBLISHING.CO*. AA- America Anywhere Buy/Sell and other services online.

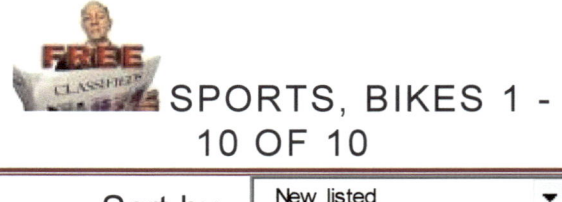

SPORTS, BIKES 1 - 10 OF 10

Sort by | New listed ▼

Taekwondo Oh Do Kwan Master Uniform

Dae Do Master Uniform in excellent condition Size 1 (would suit 11-13 year old).

sports, bikes2 weeks ago

$55

Bianchi camaleonte sport hybrid road bike

This is a 2013 Bianchi Camaleonte Sport 2 (Due) hybrid bike. Was purchased in Oct 2013 and has covered no more than 100 miles. As can be expected from a premium bicycle brand like Bianchi it has full Shimano Alvio...

sports, bikes30 weeks ago

$300

Custom Merida Big nine Carbon XT Edition

2013 Big Nine Carbon dual suspension XC bike size Medium 17 inch Less than 12 months old serviced by BNG in Townsville Selling due to change in style of bikes looking to go a carbon hardtail for 2014 Upgrades Include...

sports, bikes0 sec

$2500

Bench Press

Condition: newIn new condition as picture,no weights included,firm price only

sports, bikes0 sec

$150

power ranges cat class 16 inch

This is a Power Ranger cat clash 16 inch tires training wheels great shape any questions email me.

sports, bikes0 sec

$15

Trek 930 Single-Track mountain bike

Trek 930 for sale, full specs here: http://bikepedia.com/QuickBike/BikeSpecs.aspx?Year=1994&Brand=Trek&Model=930&Type=bike#.Ur4Ywn-9KSM Cost over 550 in 1994, clean, solid black frame, these USA made bikes will last forever. 18in frame fits 5'7-6ft. Upgraded Bontrager 26in slick/city tires

sports, bikes0 sec

$150

Small frame ladies bike with child seat

Used this as a station bike.

$25

Can use a tune up but can ride as it. Baby seat is an older model and small, would not fit anyone bigger than 2 years sports, bikes0 sec

21 Speed Diamondback Peak

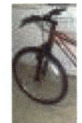

It's a small frame so you would have to be shorter than 5'6" to ride this bike. Has front and under the seat shocks and smooth street tires. Good condition. sports, bikes0 sec

$60

Fuji Classic Track Bike

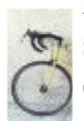

Fuji Classic 61cm Track Bike. Used, but in great shape. Includes the original drop handlebars with secondary brake leavers added. Also, new Odyssey pedals. sports, bikes0 sec

$400

Fuji Palisade 12 speed 65 CM

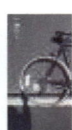

Please leave a number if you email me. Mint condition, tuned, greased and ready to ride with a 25" frames. sports, bikes0 sec

$280

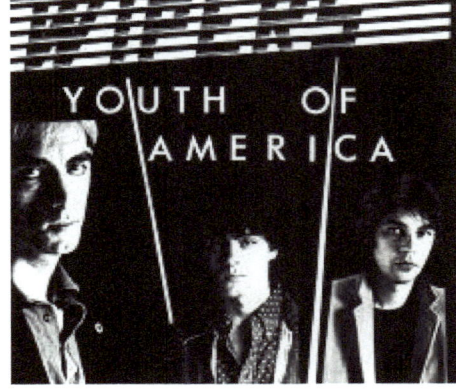

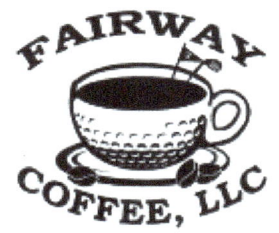

75 cents off purchase of Sunrise Bagel product

75 cents off purchase of Sunrise Bag...

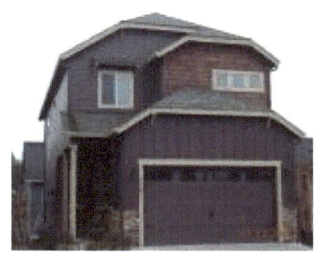

3703 NW 122ND ST Vancouver WA 98685

$296,000 MLS #:14132612
Bedrooms: ...

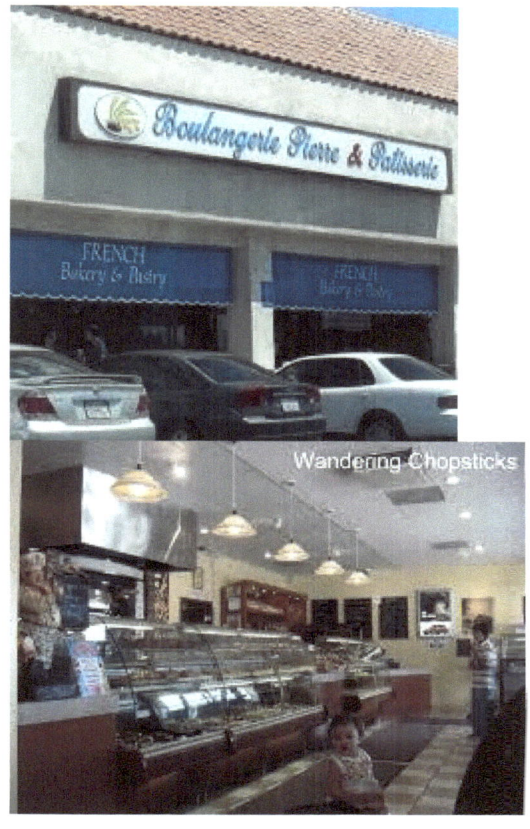

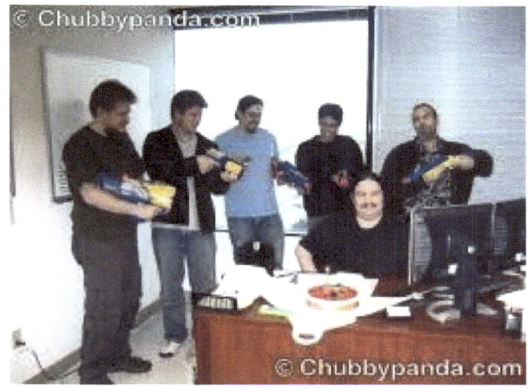

BOULANGERIE PIERRE &
PATISSERIE - GARDEN
GROVE, CA

14352 Brookhurst St, Garden Grove, **CA** 92843.

LITTLE SAIGON

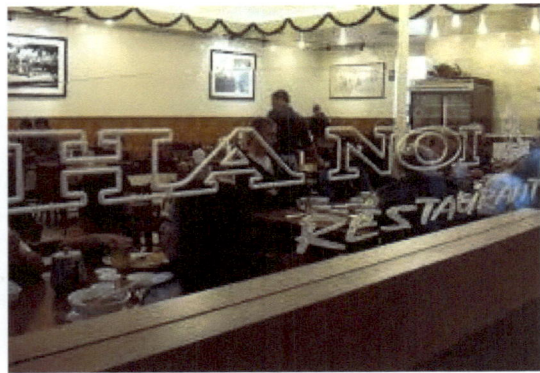

Ha Noi Restaurant – Westminster | gas

gastronomyblog.com576 × 11 Search by image

December 23, 2007. Cuisine: Vietnamese. 9082 Bolsa Avenue Westminster, CA 92683. Phone: 714-901-8108. Website: http://www.hanoirest.com/index.html

HI-CREST LIQUOR & JUNIOR MARKET

- **12055 Chapman Ave**
- Get Directions
- Phone number(714) 971-5463

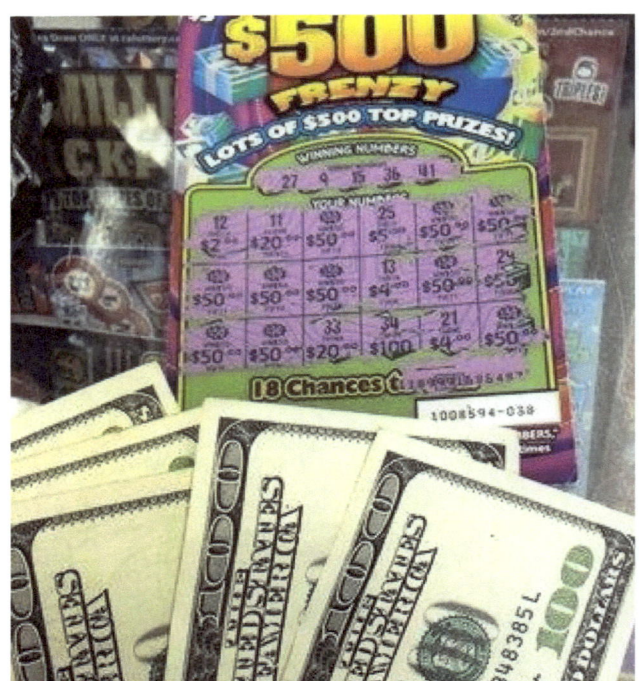

Winners are sold here!

Winners are sold here!

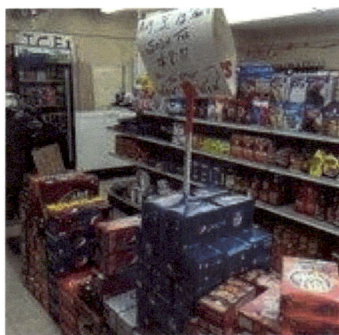

ANY 12 pack 3 for 9

ANY 12 pack 3 for 9

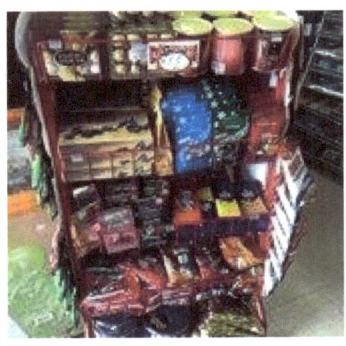

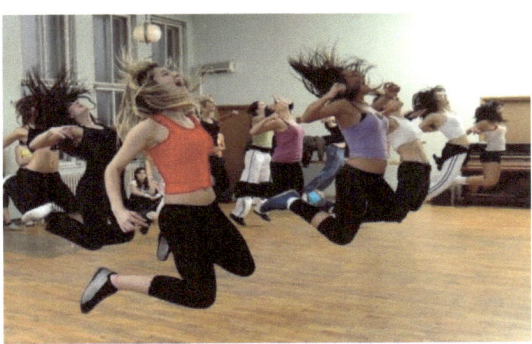

FITNESS FUN DANCE AND MORE. ZUMBA FITNESS JOIN THE PARTY WITH STUDIO B IN GARDEN GROVE AT WEST STREET AND CHAPMAN AVE NEXT TO CERTIFIED MARKET CALL FOR DIRECTION AND CLASS SCEDULE OR VISIT US..714 269-0411..ZUMBA STUDIO B JOIN THE FUN PARTY. FITNESS AND MORE.. Garden Grove 12046 West Street Garden Grove, California 92840 7 Get Directions $5 PER CLASS OR $35 PER MONTH

Great holiday deals! Only at hi crest!

ZUMBA FITNESS DANCE, JOIN THE PARTY, FUN AND MORE. $5 PER CLASS OR $35 ENTIRE MONTH OF ZUMBA. Garden Grove 12046 West Street Garden Grove, California 92840 714-269-0411 Get DirectiONS

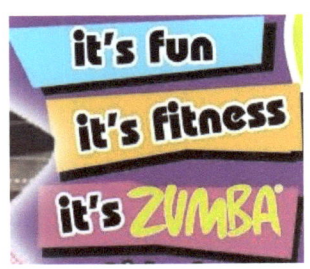

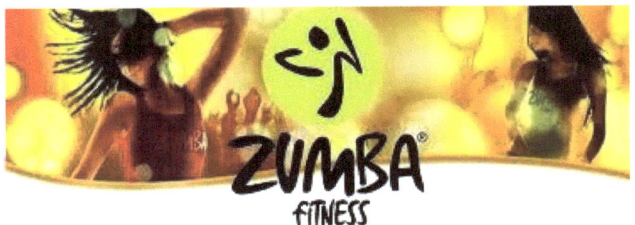

www.ingramcontent.com/pod-product-compliance
Lightning Source LLC
Chambersburg PA
CBHW041504280526
45792CB00004B/1122